Profile of a Top-Ranked School of Nursing

Mabel A. Wandelt, PhD, RN, FAAN
Professor Emeritus

Mary E. Duffy, PhD, RN
Assistant Professor

Susan E. Pollock, PhD, RN
Assistant Professor

School of Nursing
The University of Texas at Austin

Pub. No. 41-1990

12248

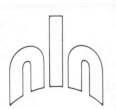

Prepared for the National League for Nursing

Printed in the United States of America
ISBN 0-88737-203-1

CONTENTS

FOREWORD

The Foundation Advisory Council of the School of Nursing of The University of Texas at Austin is composed of private citizens; its primary function in behalf of the school is to seek private funding for specific purposes. When the council requested information about other schools of nursing, the purpose was to use comparisons to identify areas needing changes in our school for which council members might seek resources. The request led to the initiation of a study that has yielded a comprehensive description of the workings of a top-ranked school of nursing. The study's results will benefit not only an advisory council needing information to support fund raising or one school planning change, but various constituencies of all schools of nursing as well.

The report is presented in the form of descriptions of the many elements and their interactions that compose the amalgam that is a top-ranked school of nursing. It provides bases for innumerable comparisons of components of any one school with those of the prototype of a top-ranked school. Those who use the information will find identified here the many and diverse persons, things, and processes functioning in a school of nursing. The information about their interactions and functioning provides descriptions of ways of implementing programs, ideas for new programs, and different ways of doing things.

If "imitation is the sincerest form of flattery," students, faculties, and administrators of the seven participating schools may view such flattery with the satisfaction of knowing that their contributions may lead to program improvements in many schools of nursing. The School of Nursing of The University of Texas at Austin is happy to provide a new basis for under-standing and emulation of processes for pursuing excellence in nursing education.

-- Dean Billye J. Brown, EdD, RN
La Quinta Centennial Professor in Nursing
School of Nursing
The University of Texas at Austin

ACKNOWLEDGMENTS

There is only one way this study could have been done. We had to ask many people to give us a great deal of their time. We described our vision of what might be accomplished and, at least tacitly, promised that the contributions would have value for many persons concerned with nursing and nursing education. We have performed our tasks to the best of our abilities; now we must attempt to thank all who expressed interest in the idea and confidence in us by sharing their time, personal perceptions, and beliefs. We hope that the deans, their assistants, the faculty, and the students who participated in the study find that they can have confidence in the report, that it will be useful to themselves and others, and that it is worthy of their investment. Our first thanks goes to them.

Dean Billye J. Brown of the School of Nursing at The University of Texas at Austin would not let the idea be put aside or its execution be delayed. Her support has been sustained in all aspects of the work, including encouragement of the authors, assignment of staff for secretarial support, and assurance of needed funding. All who find the report useful are in her debt.

Work was begun on the study within days of the ideas's first being expressed. This made it necessary to seek funds from a source that could handle expeditious consideration of a request. Dr. Pamela Maraldo, Executive Director of the National League for Nursing, expressed immediate interest in the project and shared communications with Dr. Virginia Jarrett, President of NLN, to bring the request to the Board of Directors of the League. The request was for partial funding to supplement support provided by the University of Texas School of Nursing and was approved by the NLN Board of Directors in December, 1984. The National League for Nursing merits gratitude for the funding and, in addition, special appreciation for publishing the report, which ensured its availability at an early date. The authors herewith express special thanks to Dr. Maraldo; Dr. Franklin Shaffer, Deputy Director; Elaine Silverstein, Acquisitions and Development Editor; Dr. Jarrett; and the Board of Directors of the League for their confidence and diverse expressions of support.

Many members of the faculty and staff of the School of Nursing at The University of Texas at Austin made various contributions to the project. Dr. Betsy Bowman, Associate Professor, spent days in libraries exploring the history, process, and reports of ranking educational programs. Her findings provided confidence in the method we used for selecting the schools and in the potential worth of pursuing the investigation. Moreover, she obtained extensive background information about the seven schools and their parent universities. The tables presented in Chapter 1 reflect a minute portion of her findings; of greater importance was unreported background information about each school that assisted the authors in preparing for the interview visits. Thank you, Dr. Bowman.

Many secretarial and administrative staff members provided prompt and efficient assistance with the various facets of the project. Dianna Newman and Kay Stanley were charged with sustained assignments. The most surprising aspect of their work was the promptness with which tasks were completed; the most noteworthy was the excellence of the pieces they produced from the sometimes very bad copy provided them. All may be viewed as role models of the staff in a top-ranked school of nursing.

Chapter 1

THE STUDY PLAN

I never before have spent two-and-one half hours discussing
only positive things--about anything. It is really a
wonderful experience.

--Baccalaureate student,
University of Washington

The study was done to determine the makeup of top-ranked schools of
nursing, with a view to preparing descriptions of the components, interactions,
and interrelationships that compose the complex amalgam that is a top-ranked
school of nursing. The descriptions will be useful to many persons concerned
with nursing education: students, faculty members, administrators, community
supporters, and others. They provide ideas and guidance against which any
school of nursing can judge the quality of its own endeavors and identify
needed changes and the means of effecting improvements.

INTRODUCTION

Nursing education programs are an integral part of institutions of higher
education. Each year approximately 30,000 persons graduate with bachelor's,
master's, or doctoral degrees in nursing from 400 colleges and universities in
the United States (NLN Nursing Data Book, 1983). In the past, nursing educators
placed emphasis on the development and implementation of the various educational
programs of study within these schools. Currently, their concerns have shifted
to the quality of such programs.

Several attempts have been made to do comparative evaluations of the
quality of educational programs in nursing, but no completely satisfactory
method has been found. Two early studies were done by Blau and Margulies
(1974), who relied on the subjective opinions of deans, and by Miller (1977),
who looked at the relationship between academic inbreeding and the quality of
educational programs. Hayter and Rice (1979) attempted to identify outstanding educational programs in nursing by looking at the number of faculty
publications originating in various institutions in three nursing journals.
Hayter (1984) conducted another study using an expanded list of 13 nursing
journals. Chaming's (1984) updated version of the Blau and Margulies study
polled deans of schools of nursing and members of the Council of Nurse
Researchers of the American Nurses' Association to determine the 20 top
nursing schools in the United States. Ten specific factors important in the
assessment of the schools were also examined. All of these reports have one
thing in common: they are based on single or multiple discrete factors. They
fail to provide the basis for understanding what makes a quality nursing
program or for planning improvements. Precisely for this reason the
Top-Ranked Schools of Nursing (TRSN) Project was undertaken.

History of the Project

The Foundation Advisory Council to the School of Nursing of The University of Texas at Austin provided the initial impetus for the TRSN Project. During the University's Centennial Year (1983), the Council raised a considerable sum of money for the school, which took the form of endowed professorships, fellowships, and lectureships. In 1984, its goal was to raise more money. To this end, it requested that Dean Billye Brown provide them with information about comparisons between the School of Nursing and other schools of nursing throughout the United States to be used when talking with potential donors about specific needs and the impact contributions could have on programs in the school.

At the time the request was made to Dean Brown, Dr. Mabel A. Wandelt was a member of the Foundation Advisory Council. Formerly the director of the school's Center for Health Care Research and Evaluation, Dr. Wandelt had extensive experience in research. When Dean Brown asked her how the needed data could be gathered, Dr. Wandelt proposed two plans. The first plan was designed to get readily usable quantitative information for the Foundation Advisory Council. The second plan was much more ambitious: to conduct a nationwide study designed to identify factors that make up top-ranked schools of nursing in the United States. Dr. Wandelt had recently participated in conducting the Magnet Hospital Study for the American Academy of Nursing and viewed the new study as its analog. Essentially, the proposed study would do for schools of nursing what the Magnet Hospital Study did for hospitals: provide a description of the elements that constitute a high-quality program.

Two faculty researchers, Dr. Mary E. Duffy and Dr. Susan E. Pollock, joined Dr. Wandelt in the development and implementation of the study. Funding to underwrite the study costs was sought from the National League for Nursing. In January 1985, NLN awarded the School of Nursing a contract for the project. Dr. Wandelt was principal investigator and Drs. Duffy and Pollock were codirectors.

THE PURPOSE OF THE STUDY

The TRSN Project had two major purposes:

1. To determine the makeup of top-ranked schools of nursing, with a view to preparing a description of the components, along with interactions and interrelationships, that compose the complex amalgam that is a top-ranked school of nursing.

2. To publish the description, making it available to any persons interested in or associated with schools of nursing.

ASSUMPTIONS

Two major assumptions were accepted for the study:

1. The rankings cited by Chamings (1984) were judged by the project team to be as reliable a set of rankings as other currently available ones.

2. The National League for Nursing Criteria for the Evaluation of Baccalaureate and Higher Degree Programs in Nursing (1983) indicate the major elements in the makeup of schools of nursing in institutions of higher education in the United States: organization and administration, students, faculty, curriculum, and resources.

DEFINITIONS

For the purpose of the study, the following definitions were used:

School of nursing: A department, a division, a college, a school or other administrative unit in a senior college or a university that provides a program or programs of education in professional nursing leading to a baccalaureate or higher degree.

Top-ranked schools of nursing: Those 20 schools of nursing ranked by deans and nurse researchers in the study by Dr. Patricia A. Chamings entitled "Ranking the Nursing Schools," published in Nursing Outlook 32, (5) (1984), 238-239.

Organization and administration: Those factors that contribute to the overall functioning and conduct of the affairs of the school of nursing.

Faculty: Those individuals employed by the school to teach courses at the bachelor's, master's, and doctoral levels.

Students: Those individuals who are matriculated in a course of study within the school of nursing for the purpose of attaining a bachelor's, master's, or doctoral degree.

Curriculum: The organization and sequencing of courses and learning experiences that comprise the total program of study toward a degree.

LIMITATIONS

This was an exploratory descriptive study that sought to identify the constellation of variables that interact within selected top-ranked schools of nursing in the United States. Limitations include the following:

1. Selection of the participating schools derived from a study that was based on the reports of a volunteer sample of deans and members of the

ANA Council of Nurse Researchers (Chamings, 1984). Although entirely adequate for construction of the description of the composite that is a top-ranked school, the sample may not be representative of all top-ranked schools of nursing.

2. Interviews were conducted by different members of the reseach team, and individual interview styles may have varied and influenced groups differently.

3. The individuals from the schools who participated in the group interviews were not selected randomly but were chosen by their respective deans or designates.

It is further recognized that the variables that were identified as contributing to the top ranking of the selected schools of nursing were made up of perceptions of individuals responding in group discussions in the seven schools. These perceptions were undoubtedly influenced by a variety of factors, such as age, education, experience, loyalty to the institution, perceptions of others, and the length of time employed at the institution, none of which was controlled for in the study.

METHODOLOGY

Before data gathering was begun, the overall plan of the study, including the proposed instruments and procedures, was approved by The University of Texas at Austin School of Nursing's Department Review Committee under the expedited review process. The research team then randomly selected a sample of 6 schools of nursing from the 20 top-ranked schools of nursing cited by Chamings (1984). Letters were sent to the respective deans, requesting their participation in the study. Included with the letter was a set of attachments that delineated the overall purpose of the study, the responsibilities of the school, information for participants, an agenda, group participant forms, and expense forms. Copies of these attachments are displayed in Appendix A.

The final sample consisted of the following schools (their rankings are in parentheses): the University of Washington (#1), the University of Illinois (#7), Wayne State University (#8), Catholic University of America (#9), the University of Maryland (#11), and Boston University (#13). A seventh school, The University of Texas at Austin (#14), because of its availability to the research team, was used to conduct the pilot investigation. The data from the pilot site were compared to the data gained from the sample sites. Since these data were found to be comparable, the pilot site data were included in the final analysis, thus expanding the sample to seven top-ranked schools of nursing.

Tables 1, 2, and 3 display pertinent background information about the seven schools of nursing in the sample and their parent institutions.

Table 1

SELECTED CHARACTERISTICS OF PARENT INSTITUTIONS OF TOP-RANKED SCHOOLS OF NURSING

University	Year Established	Support	Library Collection* (volumes)	Medical Center
Boston University	1839	Independent	1,495,764	Yes
Catholic University of America	1887	Private (affiliated with Roman Catholic Church)	1,114,000	No
University of Illinois at Chicago	1867	State	8,426,711	Yes
University of Maryland at Baltimore	1807	State	1,729,126	Yes
University of Texas at Austin	1883	State	5,209,536	No
University of Washington	1861	State	4,296,319	Yes
Wayne State University	1868	State	1,996,618	Yes

*Source: Chronicle of Higher Education, May 15, 1985, p. 12.

Table 2

STUDENTS AND FACULTY AT PARENT INSTITUTIONS AND TOP-RANKED SCHOOLS OF NURSING

| University | Number of Full-Time Students | | Number of Full-Time Faculty | | Percentage of Faculty with Doctorates | |
	University	School of Nursing	University	School of Nursing	University	School of Nursing
Boston University	29,157	661	2,600	75	79%	29%
Catholic University of America	6,947	360	616	39	85%	46%
University of Illinois at Chicago	17,307	641	1,874	98	70%	32%
University of Maryland at Baltimore	4,682	689	1,283	126	80%	48%
University of Texas at Austin	48,039	470	2,100	63	80%	52%
University of Washington	34,468	552	2,600	85	82%	56%
Wayne State University	29,425	353	2,100	58	85%	36%

Table 3

SELECTED CHARACTERISTICS OF TOP-RANKED SCHOOLS OF NURSING

School of Nursing	Ranking*	Year Established	Current Number of Full-Time Students			Average Cost of Program per Year (BSN only)**	Number of FAANS on Faculty
			BSN	MS	Doctoral		
Boston University	13	1946	291	311	59	$8,996	3
Catholic University of America	9	1933	246	101	13	6,920	4
University of Illinois at Chicago	7	1949	441	142	58	2,724	9
University of Maryland at Baltimore	11	1889	545	130	14	1,273	5
University of Texas at Austin	14	1976	292	54	124	500	6
University of Washington	1	1945	321	194	37	1,302	23
Wayne State University	8	1945	253	74	26	2,150	6

*Source: P. A. Chamings, "Ranking the Nursing Schools," Nursing Outlook, 32, No. 6 (1984), 238–239.

**Source: Master's Education in Nursing: Route to Opportunities in Contemporary Nursing, 1984–85 (New York: National League for Nursing, 1984).

SELECTION OF GROUP MEMBERS

The research design called for small-group interviews with members of five groups that the research team judged to be the constituencies of the school of nursing:

Administration: the dean, associate and assistant deans, department chairs.

Senior faculty: full and associate professors.

Junior faculty: assistant professors and instructors.

Graduate students: master's and doctoral students.

Undergraduate students: RN and generic students.

The deans or their designates were asked to invite six members from each group to participate in the group interview. The only stipulation they were asked to follow in the selection process was that the individuals invited should be knowledgeable about the school. Each person invited was provided with a copy of the Information for Participants form (Appendix A), which assured them that participation in the study was voluntary and that their choice not to participate in the study would not hurt their relations with the school.

GROUP INTERVIEW PROCESS

A modification of the focus-group interview was used for data collection. The technique was suggested by Billye J. Brown and developed by Mabel Wandelt for the 1980 study, Conditions Associated with Registered Nursing Employment in Texas and used for the American Academy of Nursing 1983 study, Magnet Hospital: Attraction and Retention of Professional Nurses. It provides an efficient and relatively inexpensive means of collecting a large quantity of data from a number of persons in a limited period of time. Perceptions, observations, and ideas expressed by various members of the group serve as stimuli to other members, who in consequence provide a larger quantity and variety of data than would be obtained through use of a more time-consuming process of individual interviews.

Two research team members conducted the five 2-hour group interviews in each of the seven schools. For each interview, one researcher served as interviewer and the other served as recorder. The interview responses were recorded only in penned notes in the recorder's own long- and shorthand. Experience with earlier use of the technique, when tape recording was done in addition to the written recordings, demonstrated that ample and relevant data were gathered by the recorder. To ensure adequate data collection in the current study, two persons served as recorders during the pilot interview and at the first school visited. The responses captured by the two recorders during all interviews matched in content, tone, and detail. Responses might have been recorded by tape recorder or stenotype, but preparation for analysis of the data would have been time-consuming and costly, whereas the data as penned by the recorder were ready for the first step in organization as soon as the interview was completed. Collecting the responses as notes penned by a recorder is the optimum process for data collection with the small-group interview technique used in this study.

The group interview proceeded in the following manner. The interviewer introduced the research team to the participants, described the study briefly, and then formally invited each of the persons to participate in the study. Each person was given two copies of the Participant Consent form (Appendix B). All were asked to sign one copy as their indication of willingness to participate and then pass the form to the recorder, who would witness it. Once the consents were completed, each participant was given a copy of the Interview Schedule (below and Appendix C). The interviewer then explained that each person would have an opportunity to respond to each of the questions on the schedule. She explained that following an initial response by the individual to whom the question was addressed, others should feel free to enter into discussion of the question. They might elaborate on the response already given or add new facets for consideration. After a period of discussion, the interviewer would ask a second person to respond to the question. She asked that each individual in turn, when asked to give a direct response, give the response that she would have given had she been the first person to respond to the question. As the interview proceeded, different individuals would be asked to be first respondent to successive questions.

One further instruction was provided as guidance for the respondents. They were reminded that the purpose of the study was to gather information that would serve as a basis for a description of the amalgam that is a top-ranked school of nursing. The plan was to identify the components in existing top-ranked schools that might be credited as contributing to the ranking. They were asked to limit their discussion to the components that they perceived as contributing to that ranking. They were asked not to propose elements that were lacking or that detract from the top ranking. In other words, they were asked to discuss the positive elements of their school.

The process of question, response, and discussion was followed until each person had an opportunity to give a direct response to each question. The group recorder monitored the time in order to make sure that each question received some attention by the group. The interviewer's role was to focus the group on the task at hand; to guide, direct, and clarify, where necessary; and to elicit as much descriptive information as possible on the topics mentioned by the group members. At least one ten-minute break was given midway during the interview.

INTERVIEW SCHEDULE

To ensure consistency in data collection from group to group within and across schools, a set of interview questions and statements was developed by the research team. (Some modifications of the schedule for future users are suggested in Appendix C.) The following nine items comprised the Interview Schedule:

1. What makes your school a top-ranked school of nursing?

2. Will you identify and describe a single aspect of your school that you consider a major element in its being cited as a top-ranked school of nursing?

3. What two or three things about your school influenced you to become a part (or remain a part) of the school?

4. What are the outstanding positive aspects about the organization and administration of your school?

5. What are the outstanding aspects about the faculty in your school of nursing?

6. What elements in the programs for students contribute to the top-ranking reputation of your school of nursing?

7. Please identify highlights of the (a) baccalaureate curriculum, and (b) the graduate curriculum in relation to:

   (1) the goals of the program(s);

   (2) the mission of the school; and

   (3) the value to students.

8. Please discuss two or three elements of resources and facilities that have major influences on the quality of the program(s) of your school.

9. Other than education of students, please describe the major social contribution of your school, including the personnel and processes that affect the contribution.

Question 1 was designed as the umbrella question. More time was allowed for its discussion than for the later questions. The rationale was to provide the spontaneity; that is, to allow group members themselves to introduce topics for discussion. The respondents had the interview schedule in hand and would have read most, if not all, of the questions during the early period of the discussions, and subsequent questions would have suggested topics to them. Nonetheless, the extended time with focus on Question 1 gave opportunity for them to introduce various topics without prompting from the interviewer. Naturally, some responses to later questions had been provided during the discussion of Question 1, but this did not detract from the usefulness of the later questions. There were always first responses from several participants that had not been introduced during the earlier discussion. Essentially, the process moved as a very animated discussion with all participants contributing their own perceptions and elaborations about those of others.

POST-INTERVIEW COMMENTS FORM

Immediately following the group interview, participants were asked to complete a written Post-Interview Comments Form (Appendix D). Whereas the interview focused on what exists in the school, the post-interview comments gave respondents an opportunity to describe their ideas of what might be. The rationale was that even before the interview most respondents would have thought of things that would improve their school. Certainly during the thinking and discussions of the interview, many would formulate ideas about means of improvement. The post-interview comments allowed them at least a limited opportunity to express these ideas; for the investigators, they provided additional information about factors contributing to a top-ranked school of nursing. The respondents spent about 30 minutes writing plans proposed as improvements for their school.

Data collection in each school took two-and-one-half days. Two group interviews were scheduled each day, and a lunch was included for the group participants of the particular day. In toto, each group spent approximately four hours with the research team. The entire data-collection period extended from the middle of December 1984 to the end of February 1985.

The data gathered from the group interviews and the post-interview written comments were carefully reviewed by the research team. Content analysis techniques were used and categories were developed, based on commonalities that emerged from the recordings of the responses. Subcategories were named to identify specifics of the major categories. The major categories and subcategories provided the framework for developing the description of the elements and their interactions and interrelationships that compose the amalgam that is a top-ranked school of nursing.

SUMMARY OF FINDINGS

There have been several published reports of studies evaluating the quality of educational programs in nursing. All have two commonalities: the evaluations are based on ratings for a single or very few discrete factors, and the information provides little or no basis for planning improvements. The current study was done to secure information about the many and varied factors contributing to the total complex that is a school of nursing. Five groups of individuals from seven top-ranked schools participated in the study. The groups were judged to be made up of persons knowledgeable about various components of the school and capable of identifying and describing their perceptions of factors that make up the progams in their schools. The report is a detailed description of the amalgam that is a top-ranked school of nursing, as constructed from the perceptions reported by 200 administrators, faculty members, and students in the seven schools of nursing. Its purpose is to provide useful information to all persons interested in U.S. schools of nursing.

A summary of the findings is necessarily limited to outlining the major contours and prominences of this profile of a top-ranked school of nursing. The profile cannot be sketched in smooth, regular contours. There is no way to identify the most important factor--there is no one thing sufficient to make a school top ranked. The narrative provides descriptions of innumerable elements and their many interactions and interrelationships that make up the composite that is a top-ranked school of nursing.

The identifiable components of a school are considered under six major headings:

Administration
Faculty
Students
Curricula
Resources
Social contribution (reputation)

Each of these components of a school has four elements: people, things, processes, and characteristics or attributes of the other elements.

The findings are presented in the body of the study as descriptions of the manner in which selected units of the four elements interact and work together to make up an identifiable component. These descriptions can be used to guide examination of any individual program or school, with a view toward identifying strengths and limitations as well as ideas for change. The descriptions focus on the people and things involved in each component and delineate the processes that they are involved with. Interspersed throughout are identification and discussion of the various characteristics and attributes that are pertinent to the people as they take part in particular processes in particular situations, or as they use things to initiate or affect processes.

This information is extensive, and just as it is impossible to identify the most important factor, it is impossible to provide a brief summary of the findings. Readers can be best served by outlines that list the elements of components ascribed to the major program areas of a school. The listings that follow identify the elements whose interrelationships and interactions are described in the narrative of the report.

ADMINISTRATION

People

    University president, vice presidents
    Dean
    Associate and assistant deans
    Department heads
    Director of centers

<u>Things for which administrators are responsible</u>

Resources and funding
Usual in school of higher education: building and space, laboratories,
faculty, equipment, libraries
Special: centers--learning, research, audiovisual, computer; faculty--
special assignment/expertise; programs
Faculty salaries, personnel, and policies
Faculty development
Curriculum
Relationships: university administration, deans
Visibility and communications
Of self, school of nursing, university
To community, state, nation, other countries
Through offices held, speaking, consultations, programs,
publications
Politics: university, state, national, nursing and health care
organizations
For school, profession, health care
Welfare of students: recruitment, scholarship and loan funds, advising

Processes

Securing needed resources
Promoting development of individuals
Involving individuals in planning; encouraging criticism and suggestions
Establishing relationship with key people in many and varied
constituencies.
Delegating responsibility
Keeping people informed: informal/formal, oral/written, etc.

Characteristics/Attributes

Honest, open, accessible, knowledgeable, visible, caring, sympathetic,
motivating, supportive, fair, imaginative, innovative, challenging,
interested, organized, systematic, accommodating, diplomatic.

FACULTY

People

Regular and visiting faculty, all ranks

Things for Which Faculty are Responsible

Instruction--strategies, materials
Curricula--plans, courses, schedules, clinical practice

Advisement
Research--student instruction, expanding knowledge base
Community service
Self-development
Professional involvement--advancement of profession
Goals and mission of school and university
Interpersonal relations--students, peers, community, agencies
Improvement of nursing care of patients
Publications

Processes

Teaching and supervising students
Participating in committee work
Conducting scientific investigations, sharing with peers and students
Consulting with staff in health care agencies
Implementing health care projects--screening, teaching, etc.
Attending workshops, seminars
Providing programs, teaching in continuing education programs
Belonging to profesional organizations, holding office, serving on
   committees and commissions
Evaluating achievements of programs, planning, and implementing changes,
   revising goals
Maintaining private clinical practice

Characteristics/Attributes

Expert, diverse, well-known, productive, energetic, enthusiastic,
   respected, supportive, innovative, empathic, caring, professional,
   committed, responsible, leadership, comprehensive, systematic,
   well-planned, organized, sharing

STUDENTS

People

Students enrolled in degree programs
   Baccalaureate--generic, RN, LVN, degree in other discipline
   Graduate--master's, doctoral

Things with Which Students are Concerned

Program
   Courses, schedules
   Study materials and sites
   Finances
   Development as professional--clinical practice, professional and
      student organizations, research

Processes

   Studying and learning
   Interacting with faculty, seeking advising
   Providing care for patients
   Using library, learning center, computers, skills laboratory
   Serving on committees--school, student organization, community program
      planning and implementation
   Planning, implementing, sharing research projects
   Socializing--peers, faculty, agency staffs
   Interacting--peers, faculty, agency staff, patients and families
   Promoting activities of student and professional organizations

Characteristics/Attributes

   Bright, independent, self-motivated, innovative, confident, assertive,
      sharing, competitive/cooperative, enthusiastic, caring, leadership,
      diligent, comprehensive, exploring, appropriate, varied (age, education,
      experience, goals, ethnicity, nationality, residence)

CURRICULA

People

   Administrators, faculty, students, community and agency members, staff of
      school of other areas in university

Things

   Bachelor's, master's, doctoral programs at main campus and off-campus sites
   Continuing education programs
   Statement of philosophy
   Program goals for each program
   Terminal objectives of each program
   Course syllabi
   Class schedules
   Clinical practicum assignments
   Clinical agencies utilized
   Evaluation plan
   Resources for the conduct of student research

Processes

   Developing
   Implementing
   Evaluating
   Revising
   Expanding

Characteristics/Attributes

Excellence and quality of program; independence and autonomy; variety of options; individualized student programs; definite structure; flexibility of structure; attainment of goals; strong clinical emphasis; integrated content; expert faculty teachers; qualified agency preceptors; highly motivated and qualified students; high expectation; strong faculty-student relationships; commitment to continual evaluation in order to improve; commitment to provision of education to various populations in need; curricular emphases on critical thinking, independent nursing judgment, professionalism, application of theory to practice, and relationships of theory, research, and practice.

RESOURCES

People

Administrators, faculty, students, community and agency members, faculty and staff of other schools and departments of university

Things

Funds
Clinical agencies and facilities
Library
University
Learning center
Research center
Computers
Plant
Equipment
Laboratories
Other schools and departments of university
Alumni association
Advisory councils
Community--other universities and schools, professional and health care organization, foundations.

Processes

Budgeting
Program planning
Collaborating
Ordering, maintaining, dispensing supplies and equipment
Planning and assigning space
Scheduling
Communicating
Negotiating

Establishing and maintaining relationships
Evaluating and accounting
Exploring, seeking, begging

Characteristics/Attributes

Adequate, up-to-date, convenient, available, accessible, usable, well-planned, generous of time and knowledge, well-stocked and supplied, comfortable, pleasant, systematic, periodic

SOCIAL CONTRIBUTION AND REPUTATION

People

Administrators
Faculty
Students
Alumni
Faculty and students of other schools

Things

Elementary and secondary schools
Hospitals
Clinics
Community groups and programs
Nursing and health care organizations
Programs of health promotion, care, and education
Courts

Processes

Developing/implementing programs for health care and promotion
Providing health care services
Coordinating health care programs in the community
Teaching
Demonstrating
Consulting: local, regional, national, international
Holding office in professional and health care organizations
Participating in political activities
Lobbying
Writing, speaking, telephoning

Characteristics/Attributes

Committed, humanistic, caring, sharing, independent, innovative, knowledgeable, competent, diplomatic, respected, well-known, leadership, enthusiastic, energetic, cooperative

REFERENCES

Blau, P.M., & Margulies, R.Z. (1974, Winter). "The reputations of American professional schools." Change, 42-45.

Chamings, P.A. (1984). "Ranking the nursing schools." Nursing Outlook, 32, 238-239.

Chronicle of Higher Education, May 23, 1985, p. 11 (Research Libraries).

The college blue book, 19th ed., narrative description (1983). New York: Macmillan.

Criteria for the evaluation of baccalaureate and higher degree programs in nursing (1983). 5th ed. New York: National League for Nursing.

Hayter, J. (1984, November/December). "Institutional sources of articles published in 13 nursing journals." Nursing Research, 357-362.

Hayter, J., and Rice, P. (1979). "Institutional sources of articles published in the American Journal of Nursing, Nursing Outlook, and Nursing Research." Nursing Research, 28, 205-209.

The insider's guide to the colleges, 10th ed. 1984-85 (1984). New York: Congdon & Weed.

McClure, M.L., Poulin, M.A., Sovie, M.D., & Wandelt, M.A. (1983). Magnet hospitals: Attraction and retention of professional nurses. Kansas City, MO: American Nurses' Association.

Miller, M.H. (1977). "Academic inbreeding in nursing." Nursing Outlook, 25, 172-177.

NLN nursing data book 1982: Statistical information on nursing education and newly licensed nurses (1983). New York: National League for Nursing.

Wandelt, M.A. et al. (1980). Conditions associated with registered nurse employment in Texas. Austin, TX: School of Nursing, University of Texas at Austin.

Chapter 2

ADMINISTRATION

Elements of administration--persons, actions, resources--were discussed extensively by students, faculty, and administrators alike, as they delineated factors that contribute to the quality of the school of nursing.

SUPPORT

Support from University

Being part of a renowned university is an important factor in a school of nursing's achieving a top ranking. A major element of the association is the support provided by the top administration of the university. Support is provided in the form of physical resources, including buildings, equipment, and library. There is academic support: curricula are carefully examined, rationales are listened to, consultation is provided to ensure the school's congruence with university educational policies and programs, approval is given for faculty recommendations, new programs are given empathetic considera-tion and approval. The school is treated with equity in budget and resources allocations and is encouraged to seek faculty of the highest quality and to add faculty members as new expertise is needed. There is support for nurse faculty to achieve tenure and promotion to full professor rank. Nurse faculty serve on university committees and are elected to chair those committees. The dean is accorded the same respect and charged with the same responsibilities for the school and the university as deans of all other schools. The board of regents, the president, and the vice-presidents know about the school of nursing and hold it in high esteem; they know its programs and goals. Top administrators have confidence in the dean and the faculty; they encourage excellence, and when a program proposal is presented to them, they ask, "What do you need to do it?" They request the participation of nurse faculty in policy decisions and program planning pertinent to the functioning of the total university. The school of nursing is an integral part of the university, and top administration supports it accordingly.

Support for Faculty Activities and Interests

Innovation is encouraged in such areas of faculty interest as research, clinical practice, new course development, and teaching strategies. Assis-tance and support are provided from persons on all levels of administration. Department chairs not only offer suggestions but also frequently become active participants in projects initiated by faculty. Assistant deans share explora-tions of ideas and assist in securing the resources needed to carry out pro-jects. They contribute greatly in securing funding, space, equipment, student assistants, and negotiated time.

Faculty describe the nature of the dean's support:

> The dean is very creative in using resources well; there are funds to support small projects, program presentations, travel, computer searches.

> Even in times of stringent budget there is funding for the research center, where faculty get assistance with research and writing.

> The dean encourages you to do whatever you want. She is also astute in picking out your talents.

> The dean provides prompt feedback; never have to wait for decisions; can make mistakes, yet be supported.

> The dean creates a supportive atmosphere for junior administrators to pursue their administrative tasks and function in their teaching and clinical roles.

> The degree of trust of the dean in the faculty is very high, and that promotes creativity and productivity in the faculty.

Conditions are conducive to scholarly productivity. Faculty teaching loads allow for great flexibility. The members of a department can plan variations in loads over several semesters. Individual faculty members are helped to plan for engagement in teaching, research, writing, and community work in various concentrations in successive semesters. They are helped to negotiate with colleagues and administration for teaching and other academic assignments. The flexibility in use of time promotes faculty productivity, both in the work of the educational program and in their own research and self-development. Assignments are negotiated with the assistant dean in collaboration with the department chairperson, and for the most part they remain constant unless a faculty member requests a change. Occasionally, individuals are encouraged to seek changes for promotion of their own professional development, to broaden their horizons and stretch the use of their potential capabilities. One faculty member comments:

> They demand a lot of us, but they help us achieve it. They don't ask us to punch a clock, and that makes a great difference in how you feel about the hours you devote to teaching and study. You have a greater feeling of working toward your own goals.

Faculty Development

There is a dual reason for the dean to give high priority to promoting faculty development: full achievement for each individual, and fulfillment of responsibility of the school to have a faculty of high academic attainment. The dean expresses the first purpose by means of continual communication and interaction with faculty members in groups and on an individual basis. For the second, she uses frequent occasions to remind the faculty of the history of nursing's involvement in universities and concomitant involvement as a scholarly, science-based profession. Early in the twentieth century, universities opened their doors to nurses, after pleas from nurse pioneers who promised that, given the opportunity to learn from scholars and associate with them in academe, nursing would develop its own cadre of scholars to take their rightful place among other disciplines in institutions of higher education. The movement toward development of scholars and of an identifiable science base for meeting the profession's obligations to society has gained momentum in the past two decades. Nonetheless, compared to many other disciplines, nursing still has a smaller proportion of faculty members who hold doctoral degrees and still lags in the volume of new knowledge being provided through research. Essentially, nursing must press forward with continual effort to advance the qualifications of its faculty and the volume and quality of its research. Commitment and activities toward these ends are conspicuous in a top-ranked school of nursing.

Faculty members comment on examples of concern and support for faculty development:

> Administration goes out of its way to support growth and development of faculty, via leaves, scheduling, and workload.

> There is open pressure and support for faculty to get the doctorate, if they do not have one. There is flexibility so that you can teach in undergraduate programs and be enrolled in a doctoral program.

> I had not considered doing a doctorate until coming here. Never thought of it; now I have made a commitment; I shall go forward.

> The various resources I need to advance professionally are here, and in addition, support and encouragement.

> The dean encourages us to research and engage in various forms of continuing education.

> Administration helps us plan each year's objectives. The dean invites us to meet with her individually to discuss career goals.

> The requirements for achieving tenure are given to us in writing during early orientation, but the dean discusses these with us in later individual conferences, and helps us plan our own progression toward tenure.

> There is support from the dean; she is always available, many times without a long-time appointment.

> Sometimes faculty can be a threat to the dean; there is none of that here. The dean wants faculty to succeed; she does not hold people back.

> The chair of my department developed a plan for my academic life, so that I had time to get my research going, to get adjusted to the new environment. There is a commitment of the school to support development of new faculty.

Administration encourages and supports faculty's scholarly endeavors. Quite satisfying to have your abilities recognized.

There is a highly qualified faculty, but they do not hesitate to take new faculty without teaching experience. There are planning and programs in place to develop new faculty, and accommodations will be made to assist individuals in their development.

Mutual Support, Respect, Recognition

Brief comments of faculty members best describe the mutual support, respect, and recognition experienced by faculty:

There is a dedication of faculty, students, staff, and administration. Administration and faculty give support when issues arise.

We receive strong encouragement from the dean and department administrators. Colleagues help us do extra things--efforts add up to more than 100 percent.

There is support through collaboration, which provides assurance of opportunity to meet goals.

I get feedback from the dean and assistant deans that I am making a contribution to the school--very important.

There is support from peers and administration; they take real pride in what we do.

We have positive reinforcement for achievement, from the dean, peers, and students.

Monetary rewards are not great, but the dean and administrators are very liberal with praise. The dean always sings praises of us in public.

Obviously, faculty appreciate expressions of respect and recognition from all with whom they work; they view the expressions as being an important element in the composition of a well-functioning school.

THE DEAN

Honest, Open, Accessible

When discussion focuses on faculty there are comments about faculty's being the primary element in the composite that is a top-ranked school. When administration is the focus, there is universal agreement that the dean is the key ingredient. The dean appreciates the confidence placed in her; she credits faculty for the program of excellence. She cites their enthusiasm, competence, and commitment in using effectively the resources, guidance, and atmosphere she is able to provide. The dean acknowledges the work of the first dean and other deans who have gone before her; she describes components of the program structure and relationships developed in the university and in the community that provide the foundation for the current programs and allow for their continuing expansion and excellence.

The dean is described by faculty and students alike as being accessible: "She is approachable as a person. There are channels, but she has an open-door policy and is always accessible." They feel comfortable going to her to discuss any topic, a new idea, a problem, a plan. She will listen and provide ideas, she will assist with solutions. There are repeated expressions that the dean "really cares" and that she knows students and is aware of strengths of individuals.

The dean is a persuasive recruiter; people are comfortable with her.

She respects faculty opinions; has an open mind; and follows through on promises. She is magnanimous in acceptance of people.

I can go to the dean and talk openly. If I can be convincing, the changes do begin to occur, and that is important.

The dean uses important leadership strategies: for example, she promotes collegiality among faculty and gives consideration to all proposals for change and promptly moves to implement improvements. She provides descriptions and rationales for the mission, philosophy, and programs of the school that convince administration of the need for continuation of the school's autonomy. She uses political savvy to secure resources and support for the school from the university administration, from the council of deans, and from legislative and governmental bodies. The dean's actions and demeanor portray her as a knowledgeable and honest person who cares very much about people.

Expert Administrator

The dean is a qualified administrator in relation to both educational background and experience. She continues to increase her knowledge and competence through seminars, work conferences, and consultation. She shares the experiences with faculty, particularly the services of visiting consultants, to enhance faculty knowledge about administration and to help them understand administration practices, policies, and rationales within the school. She urges faculty to offer suggestions for the running of the school and for improvements. She knows the gamut of responsibilities of a chief executive officer; she devotes needed attention, time, and effort to fulfilling the responsibilities and makes judicious use of staff and faculty in needed activities and programs. She seeks well-qualified persons for each position and assists all to increase their competence at assigned responsibilities.

Among her top-priority responsibilities is the securing of funding, not only for the usually recognized teaching programs but also for special requirements, such as the centers for learning and research, computers, support of faculty research and travel, and student scholarships and loans. She seeks funds for special projects of individual faculty members. A second priority is for faculty development; she devotes time and effort to promoting programs for groups and for individuals, including lengthy planning and supportive conferences with individuals. She is a motivator who uses all available means to challenge faculty members: an invitation to discuss career planning, notes reminding individuals of particular meetings, loan of a journal article, questions about outcome of latest planned activities, and others. One faculty member commented, "The dean is so interested and supportive that one would have to really want to fail, not to succeed."

The dean is good at reading and responding to political forces. She has functioned during changes of the university president and various vice-presidents and has managed to advance the causes of the school with each of them.

The dean fully understands all programs and willingly discusses ideas or problems about them with any concerned individual, including students. She wants to know students and makes sure that students are involved in all appropriate committees in the school and that they participate with voice and vote.

Another area of responsibility of the dean that was frequently mentioned by the faculty and sometimes by students is the development and maintenance of working relationships with community agencies. Of primary concern are the agencies where students have clinical experiences, but there are many other types of agencies with whom relationships must be kept functional. They include organizational and community groups that might be interested in providing financial support for programs or students, community groups and programs for whom the faculty and students might provide unique services, and political groups and individuals who influence laws pertinent to health care and professional practice. The dean must know key people in these organizations and must be aware of their programs so that communications, programs, and activities can be promoted to the mutual benefit of the agencies and the school. Further, she must encourage faculty members, students, and alumni to maintain contact with many agencies.

Workload

For a dean, a major administrative responsibility is establishing faculty workload, which in turn is closely tied to planning and support for faculty development. Comments of the dean and faculty describe the situation:

> As an administrator, research is the number 1 priority. Time gets set aside; depending on rank, there is usually one day a week. Greatest thing we have done; it costs money, but it is worth it.

> We keep reasonable teaching loads, using a working formula of a 2:4:6 ratio. In PhD program, 1 faculty for 2 students; MS, 1:4; BSN, 1:6.

> Good faculty-student ratio. Students get a lot of special attention and faculty are not bogged down.

Conditions are conducive to scholarly productivity. Generally, faculty members negotiate with department head for workload, done on an individual basis. This is a great strength.

New faculty get highest priority for TA assistance, which is done to give them to do their research.

We have one day a week as a research day. Work wherever it serves us: at home, library, or elsewhere. There is no time-clock punching.

We are not overloaded clinically. Care is shown in planning workloads.

Faculty have a fairly light lecture load, which gives opportunity to promote our professional growth in other areas.

Course assignments are approaching what is being done in major universities; they are assigned primarily according to individual expertise.

We use team teaching in our department (ten hours of theory per semester), plus two days a week in clinical. We can use our time for other activities.

Faculty are not overworked--teach one or two courses per semester. Have time for student conferences and their other faculty responsibilities. They are not hassled.

Advisory Groups

The dean maintains several formal advisory groups. There is a faculty committee composed of professors of all rank, with some appointed by the dean and some elected by the faculty for staggered two-year terms. This committee advises the dean in all faculty personnel matters. It plays a major role in delineating faculty qualifications for employment and promotions and develops materials for faculty evaluations and implements and monitors that program.

A second advisory committee is made up of the director of nursing and student coordinator of each of the health-care facilities that are used for clinical experiences of students. Chairpersons of the departments in the school are also members of this committee. The committee meets twice a year. In late summer, the dean presents the planning for the coming year, and schedules for students and for the agency staffs are reconciled. At the late spring meeting, the largest input is from the staffs of the agencies. They report their experiences with the student instructional program during the year being completed and make suggestions for planning for the following year. These two half-day meetings mark a major collaborative effort, which is supplementary to the communications between agency staffs and faculty that take place throughout the academic year.

A third advisory group is established to communicate with and involve the larger community in the concerns of the school. The dean establishes an advisory committee of persons who have particular interests in the school.

They include retired nurses, physicians and physicians' spouses, hospital administrators, interested citizens, and others. They are organized into a formal structure, with an executive committee and active working committees, each composed of advisory committee members and others and chaired by a committee member. The larger committee meets in the school at least twice a year; working committees meet more frequently, as needed. The primary purpose of the advisory committee is to secure funds to be used to promote the programs of the school. During the semiannual meetings the members learn details about the school program and progress. They plan for promotional activities. The finance committee outlines the needs of the school and plans fund-raising activities. Throughout the year, committee members work individually, in teams, and in collaboration with the dean and the liaison from the university development office to identify and communicate with individuals and representatives of foundations, organizations, and businesses to inform them about the school's programs and needs, the ways in which funds would be used, and how funds would be handled by the school and the university. The process in recent years has yielded hundreds of thousands of dollars that have been used to endow professorships, support visiting lectures, provide scholarships and loans for students, and provide equipment for particular projects. The advisory committee has greatly broadened the community of the school, particularly the community that knows about the school of nursing and its programs and that makes positive contributions to the implementation of those programs.

Relationships with University Administration, Other Deans, and Others on Campus

Top university administrators know that the school has received national recognition for the quality of its programs. They view the dean as a leader among the deans and rely on her for contributions to the total university. Other deans respect her; seek her counsel and support; and are liberal in sharing knowledge, planning, and support with her. She has good relations with deans of health-related schools--pharmacy, medicine, allied health, and public health. There is sharing among the schools, with particular focus on needs of students for courses, laboratory facilities, libraries, and research resources, including access to patients. Besides having personal and administrative clout that makes it possible to get things for the school, the dean is continually enlarging the circle of individuals within the university with whom she maintains friendly and professional relationships. As a result, the school of nursing takes an ever more integral part in the university organization, to the benefit of the faculty and students, the university, and the community.

Dean's Style

Brief comments from faculty members and students portray the dean's style:

The dean's administrative style is very loose, but supportive.

The dean is positive, confirming, and affirming. I had an article accepted and she took me to lunch. We were both very busy, but she wanted me to know how happy she was for me.

Both in individual conversations and in group meetings, the dean communicates challenge and stimulation. The communication is frequently so subtle that you are not aware of the message for days, but the ideas and the hints are there, and they will come up again, accompanied by encouragement and support.

The dean sets the tone. She is visible in nursing circles and encourages faculty to be visible. Things are happening here; she is a great influence on faculty.

The dean encourages faculty independence. She is willing to help.

Notices of congratulations to individuals for achievements are posted on the bulletin board outside the dean's office.

Administration is open to students; the dean is interested in them and always available. She is just like anyone else.

Reputation of the Dean

The dean has a local, national, and international reputation as a leader in professional nursing and an educational administrator with outstanding knowledge and skills. She has held high elective office in most major state and national nursing organizations. She influences the image of nursing held by nurses, allied health professionals, legislators, community leaders, and consumers. She has extensive visibility, which continues to grow as she accepts national committee and commission assignments and speaking engagements. She is ever ready to inform people about the university, the school, and particular programs and persons in the school.

One faculty member commented, "She is respected and admired outside the school. She is a major reason for my coming here, and I continue to be increasingly happy that she represents us." Some faculty members believe that the dean's reputation precedes that of the school and its programs and that it is the initial force in the recruitment of international students and students from other states.

The dean not only administers competently but also she writes about what she knows best; she publishes articles about various facets of nursing educational administration in journals that reach nurses with varied interests. Besides informing about administration of educational programs, the articles describe a major concern of the administrator: caring about students and faculty. There are articles deriving from her own investigations into problems of varied concern to nurses and nurse educators; problems relating to sciences, teaching, and nursing care of patients. That the dean's reputation extends beyond the immediate community and the field of nursing is evidenced by awards from state and national groups with large community involvement, such as state woman of the year, regional leading woman educator, and outstanding educator of America. The dean is known nationally and internationally. Among the attributes composing her reputation are creativity, innovativeness, energy, and willingness to listen, to talk, and to travel.

Concern for Students

The dean and other administrators are open to students, interested in them, and always accessible to them.

> The dean teaches the first course in nursing: sets the stage, focus, and attitudes for students toward the program and nursing.

> Students feel complimented that she would do this. The class removed all doubts that I had about opting for nursing; I know now I made the right choice.*

The dean is attuned to students; she knows their strengths and weaknesses and encourages creativity and innovation in them. She fosters a personal relationship with them by attending student-sponsored social functions and by hosting annual receptions for various groups of students. A student declared, "I even know the dean and she has a sense of humor."

The dean supports flexibility in programs to accommodate needs and interests of individual students. Older students find this particularly meaningful. Many of them have well-formulated goals that they hope to achieve through the nursing program; others need accommodations in scheduling because of commuting or family requirements. When students discuss the dean, they speak of the quality of the education they are receiving. Comments of two students express student perceptions:

> They're not pumping out nurses here. They're more interested in the quality of the product than in producing numbers.

> The dean impresses us with the fact that we are professional and we have to behave and practice as professionals. There is so much more involved in nursing than I ever thought. I, as a student, realize I can make a difference.

Students credit the dean with making it possible for them to fulfill their individual potentials. They view the dean as a role model for faculty and for students who subtly inspires them to want to be exemplary nurses and to have confidence in their abilities and satisfaction in their attainments.

---

*Student of Dean Rheba de Tornyay, University of Washington.

ORGANIZATIONAL STRUCTURE

Departments and Committees

The organizational structure is fairly complex, but essentially it is composed of departments charged with implementing instructional programs and committees charged with curriculum and program planning, policymaking, and overseeing student and faculty personnel matters. The faculty members see the various components of structure as strengths. Although structure is well-defined, there is a free flow of communications across department lines, which promotes functioning of committees. Committees have appointed and elected members, and most have student representatives. No-protest voting is a mechanism used effectively to expedite communication and enhance the quality of committee decisions and recommendations. All faculty members can have input into all decisions, yet they do not have to spend time in meetings of the whole faculty in order to make suggestions. The faculty like the fewer meetings, the more effective committee obligations, and the time for other things.*

Faculty members express satisfaction with the functioning of the organizational structure and the opportunity it gives them to be involved in the governance of the school:

> The department and committee structures are positive aspects that allow us to manage issues and get the work done.

> Issues are handled well within departments.

> There is extensive faculty input into decision making and policy-making; the dean solicits suggestions about administrative policy.

> There is tremendous freedom within the school; the faculty have input into their own destiny; and the structure helps faculty to advance their own initiatives.

> Faculty have control over curriculum issues.

> Administration encourages suggestions for change and is willing to try things.

> Lines of authority are very clear. Faculty know them and who's responsible for what. Faculty understand and are comfortable addressing persons who assist with development of ideas and seeing them through the system.

> Everyone has input, and changes are made as needed.

---

*Described in detail at University of Texas at Austin.

Organizational structure allows for faculty input and change. The intent is to help us be stronger in our scholarly work.

Faculty are independent here and always have had a lot of input into decisions.

There is a clear separation of what is administration responsibility and what is faculty responsibility.

OPPORTUNITY TO LEARN AND TO PRODUCE

Variety of Specialty Areas

Faculty are enthusiastic about opportunities to learn and to grow. Many describe the situation as being a major reason for their coming to the school and for remaining. They speak of the variety of opportunities in terms of varied clinical and functional programs, faculty and students with varied expertise and interests, and opportunities to change and try new things. The latter may range from a short-term learning experience to a planned change in career focus. Many describe the opportunities for learning as contributing to and deriving from the exciting atmosphere. There seems to be a never-ending stream of discussions of new ideas, progress in studies, and reports of findings of research that will make a difference in nursing care.

There is opportunity to grow here; to get involved in all sorts of things. It is never boring.

People to Work With

A few brief comments by faculty members express their feelings about opportunities afforded by association with people with whom they work:

There is opportunity to work with faculty who have longstanding reputations for research.

Other faculties seek to recruit our faculty for their schools, not only with invitations, but [they] propose challenges in terms of professional responsibility to "share the wealth."

There are several annual programs that provide for visiting professors and lectures--all with national reputations.

Senior faculty are entering into mentor relationships with junior faculty.

Senior faculty are willing to share discussions about their research and welcome requests from junior faculty for assistance in their own developmental efforts.

I like being a professional scholar; as faculty here you are indeed a professional student among professional students.

Individual Growth

There is encouragement and tolerance of independent thinking and pursuit of individual ideas and interests. There is a freedom to express individual ideas and disagree with the ideas of others. Faculty members confidently seek assistance and support to advance their personal growth: teaching schedules and workload can be negotiated to allow time for study, attendance at classes and meetings, and writing. There is sharing among faculty members to accommodate colleagues' scheduling needs. Other schools in the university and other universities in the area provide varied opportunities for doctoral study.

There is planning and support for individual faculty members who pursue self-development with an eye to attaining tenure. Tenure is recognized as a high attainment, but is is viewed as only a beginning, a highlight along the course of continued growth and pursuit of learning and self-improvement. Most planning and scheduling to accommodate self-development activities for individual faculty members occurs at the departmental level. The department chairperson provides advice and counseling, and all members of the department collaborate in extended planning for fulfillment of departmental teaching responsibilities and scheduling for individual faculty. There are variations among departments and from semester to semester, but each department devotes about 40 percent of its time to research, writing, and other developmental pursuits.

Accommodations are made to support development of individual faculty members as they engage in activities pertinent to any of the three primary areas of academic responsibility: teaching, research, and community service. The general planning within a department includes reminders of the need for individuals to plan their efforts to ensure involvement and production in each of the areas. Younger faculty members receive guidance with planning so that they do not disperse their energies in attempts to cover all three areas equally at any one time. They learn to concentrate selected areas for semester- or year-long blocks of time. Two- and three-year plans are found helpful for faculty members who are learning to plan time for personal development and for full involvement in and contribution to the missions of the school and university. Plans for time to devote to nonteaching activities may include blocks of time ranging from one-half day a week, to a month during class interims, to year-long sabbaticals. Faculty members are encouraged to be imaginative in planning, and administration assists in accommodating the plans.

ADMINISTRATION'S EXPECTATIONS OF FACULTY

Continued Growth, Goal-Directed Activities

Expectations of the faculty are high. Individuals are expected to delineate goals for continued growth, with sights being set on attainment of excellence. Expectations are made clear, and there is varied and extensive support for achievement of goals. Faculty who do not hold the doctorate are expected to engage in a program of study toward the degree. Faculty know when they come to the school that they will be expected to work toward personal goals and to contribute to programs toward achieving the goals of the school. The faculty find the expectations motivating for study and involvement: "Expectations are high and rewards follow if they are met."

The dean uses the top ranking of the school as a challenge to the faculty for movement toward change and improvement. She asks, "Do we deserve to have a top ranking? Why might we not deserve it?" The challenge does not diminish the pride or confidence of the faculty; rather, it serves as stimulus for continued questioning, planning, and innovation for improvements in all facets of the program.*

Excellence

Faculty members find the expectations of personal excellence to be stimulating; they view them as evidence of confidence in their personal commitment to work toward the goals of the school. There are repeated reminders that faculty serve as role models for excellence in nursing, teaching, and research, not only for students but also for nurses in the community and for faculties in other schools. There is an elitism expressed in the standards set for teaching, research, and community service. Faculty are encouraged to engage in activities in areas of individual interests and strengths, within and outside the school. They are expected to demonstrate their competence and are supported in projects they devise for doing so.

Faculty are reminded that they are expected to engage in social and civic activities as a part of faculty responsibility. They are particularly encouraged to contribute in their individual areas of strength: leaders are expected to lead; clinicians to assist in and guide clinical practice; teachers to provide instruction to various community groups and others. The varied and extensive activities include:

-- Talks in high schools: instruction on health issues and recruitment of students for the health professions.

-- Participation in town meetings.

-- Monitoring health care legislation and providing information to legislators.

-- Serving on boards of directors of health agencies.

_____

*Credit to Dean Rheba de Tornyay, University of Washington.

-- Providing educational programs for staffs of all agencies used for student clinical practice.

-- Involving students in health care services at civic programs (for example, the county fair, rodeo, air show).

Recognition for displays of excellence is accorded by administration, colleagues, and students; all view the achievements as assets to the school and the university.

EVALUATION

Evaluation, of a sort, has always been part of the program of a school of nursing. Primary among evaluations were those of student performance. Once there were vaguely structured evaluations of faculty at the time of consideration for promotion. When national accreditation became an expectation, evaluations were done of various facets of the programs in relation to nationally established criteria. In recent years all evaluations have become more systematized and have involved many more persons in the evaluation of each program component. The self-study done for national accreditation is an occasion for comprehensive study of the programs, but this is required only at eight-year intervals. A detailed plan has now been established for more frequent evaluations, with schedules for measurement of processes of work and goal achievement of all aspects of the program required by the accreditation agency. Evaluations of various aspects of program are scheduled at varying frequencies, from annual to five-year periods. A master plan shows the elements of each program of the school that are to be evaluated: Criteria are delineated for evaluation of each discrete element to be evaluated, specific measurements to be used as evidence of the degree to which each criterion is met are spelled out, and the membership of the committee charged with responsibility for each evaluation is delineated.* The school's evaluation committee develops a specific charge and schedule for each committee and receives the committees' reports.

Evaluation of the total program of the school is a continuing program in itself; its goals are those commonly ascribed to evaluation: accounting for the work of the school and providing information on which to base requests for funds and other resources, and planning for changes, additions, improvements. The ongoing systematic evaluation program provides a current picture of the total program, in contrast to the incomplete picture that is provided when self-studies for accreditation are relied on to provide information about the status of the quality of any individual program.

Evaluation of the total program of the school is a continuing program in itself; its goals are those commonly ascribed to evaluation: accounting for the work of the school and providing information on which to base requests for

---

*The most complete plan was described at the University of Maryland.

funds and other resources, and planning for changes, additions, improvements. The ongoing systematic evaluation program provides a current picture of the total program, in contrast to the incomplete picture that is provided when self-studies for accreditation are relied on to provide information about the status of the quality of any individual program.

For evaluation of faculty, the school of nursing follows the pattern prescribed by the university administration, with periodic evaluations of individual faculty members ranging from annual evaluations for instructors and assistant professors to evaluation every five years for full professors. Evaluations that are done for tenure include evaluations from peers outside the university. Just as for the program evaluations, criteria and relevant measurements are clearly spelled out in the faculty evaluation plan. Faculty members are supplied with a copy of the plan during orientation.

Essentially, all students, staff, and faculty are involved in doing measurements and being measured in one or more evaluations. Most believe the evaluations serve a valuable purpose and should be done. Many question the need for the number of evaluations done and many would "just like to have someone else do it." Nonetheless, all acknowledge that evaluation presents the program in a positive light and has sufficient benefits to individuals and to the school to warrant the extensive work involved:

> Constant evaluations are done on every level. Everyone knows what is going on, and we have made good changes. We're not afraid to look at ourselves and make changes.

> Expectations are very clear. Evaluation process for faculty is very objective; "no game playing here."

> Faculty insist on your evaluation of courses. You won't get a grade unless you evaluate the course. Evaluations are very specific and comprehensive--from lectures to each objective. Really give active feedback.

> We separate planning for change from planning for maintenance accomplishment. What do we need to maintain our stance in top ranking? What do we need to change? We now need to devote more attention to future planning.

ORGANIZATION

Structure and Faculty Involvement

The dean provides for extensive faculty involvement in organization and administrative matters. When a major organizational change is to be made, she schedules two- to three-day retreats as a means of informing the faculty, focusing attention for concentrated and prolonged periods of time, having faculty develop new awareness about each other, and facilitating cohesion in establishing goals and planning for steps needed to achieve the goals. The dean sets up a small committee to help plan the agenda, which is fairly tight and makes considerable demands on faculty to attend to the work at hand and to cooperate so that decisions and mutually agreed-upon goals can be delineated. The retreats allow for expeditious planning for changes in structure, for reinforcement, and for commitment to implementation of programs. There is opportunity to redefine administration's role and faculty's role in executing the programs.

Essentially, the organization is simple and clear. There is a limited number of standing committees that spend limited amounts of time making decisions. It is clear which decisions must be made by administration and which must be made by the faculty. These demarcations, however, do not preclude a free flow of communication and sharing of information and opinions as decisions are made. The faculty feels that they have a high degree of personal responsibility; they know to whom they are responsible, and they are comfortable discussing issues and problems with persons on all levels of administration.

The dean relies extensively on faculty input for decisions about faculty hiring and promotion. A committee, composed of all full professors and elected associate and assistant professors, is charged with development and updating of criteria for various ranks; interviewing applicants and making recommendations to the dean; and collecting materials, reviews, and recommendations to the dean about promotions. Individual committee members assume responsibility for using semiformal and informal communications to help all faculty members understand the bases and processes of personnel decisions; in turn, the faculty views functioning of the committee as providing for faculty input into the important decisions.

The committee-departmental structure provides for decisions to be made at the lowest possible level of the structure. It is clearly understood when recommendations from faculty constitute decisions and when they are advice to a higher level, but the structure promotes faculty interest and satisfaction with participation in the running of the school.

A few comments demonstrate faculty perceptions about their involvement in decisions:

> It is a tight, yet flexible structure.

> Administration has prerogatives and faculty have prerogatives. Faculty understand the role they plan in decision making.

> I am impressed by the level of collegiality in the groups; not departmentally territorial. People share; great teamwork.

> Administration people are clear in their role; yet flexible when we need to look at goal rather than role.

> Organizational structure permits freedom to move. There are good formal and informal channels of communication.

> Faculty have opportunity for input without excessive meetings.

Stability in organization; people have been here a long time; they are stable administrators.

Students state that their knowledge of the administrative organization of the school is limited, but some of their perceptions are expressed as follows:

Not a rigid, but a structured administration. You can approach anyone; students can find out early who to go to.

The whole program is shown in the general course packet when you come. Only at end of program do you realize that all are building blocks to prepare you to be a good graduate. It runs well, so it must be OK.

You know where to go to get a problem solved. That is the ultimate and even if people change, the structure is consistent, a great time saver.

Don't have to go through a million channels to talk to somebody.

Students have an active role in the school; they are members on all standing committees and they are listened to.

Departments

The departmental structure is perceived as being a strength by both administration and faculty:

Department structure is a very positive thing here. Department heads have great latitude and leeway to develop their own specialty and sub-specialties. A pretty traditional system but with some flexibility.

Department structure makes for a strong identification with people in your field; it makes sense with a large faculty.

We have preserved clinical departments; faculty have a sense of power and they support administration.

It is a positive thing to be able to negotiate your workload and professional goal activities at department level.

The department head is a facilitator, not a dictator.

Another strength of departments is that they give everyone a home base.

Administrative structure and functioning, along with their own involvement in decisions about programs and their responsibilities for curriculum and instructional matters, obviously receive much thought and discussion by faculty members. Also, faculty members are obviously satisfied with most aspects of this complex component of the school.

ASSOCIATE AND ASSISTANT DEANS

From the dean's persepective, the faculty members in administrative positions are knowledgeable and competent administrators. They relieve her from having to handle day-to-day concerns that are important to individuals, but of limited import to the functioning of the total enterprise. The dean takes pride in a mark of an effective administration: programs go on as smoothly when she is away as when she is in the school. She has confidence in administrators' abilities to make decisions in her absence. There are good working relationships and communications among the associate and assistant deans. They are responsible for planning for changes and for making long-range projections. There is a lack of territoriality; rather, sharing, trust, and mutual respect are conspicuous in all of their deliberations, resulting plans, and suggested resource allocations.

Impressions of junior faculty about higher administration are expressed in these terms:

> Dean and associate and assistant deans work hard--excellent role models for us to work hard. They are very liberal with their praise for us.

> Personalities of the dean and top administrators make a difference.

> They present themselves as being concerned about faculty; this helps us.

> As faculty I do not have to worry about nitty-gritty. Someone else does it; I can get on with my teaching and research. Administration is approachable; don't have to trek through a trail of examiners.

Students, too, perceive the value of the deans:

> I am not aware of the organizational structure at all. I don't think of a chain of command--just go to someone, and I get needed help.

> I took for granted what was here--now in this interview, I learn that maybe there are special good things.

> Administrators are receptive to students' problems; they enjoy talking to students.

> I like separation of graduate and undergraduate programs. I go to undergraduate dean and do not have to compete with graduate students for attention.

> If I had a problem, I'd know where to take it. I'd be comfortable to approach an administrator with either a complaint or suggestion.

> I never have to talk to the dean; I can always find out what I am looking for.

The capable administrative group functions competently, effectively, and, most of all, unobtrusively, to advance programs and meet needs of all persons in the school, from undergraduate students to junior faculty to the dean.

HONESTY, TRUST

References to honesty and trust frequently enter into discussions with the faculty. There are comments about the integrity of the dean and her administrators. Faculty members remark on their reputation for keeping promises-- promises made at the time of hiring and those made during negotiations for assignments and planning for personal development and attainment of career goals. To the faculty, confidence that they are trusted to proceed along self-selected paths for accomplishing their jobs is extremely important. Administrators express their assurance of a mutual trust; they are confident that faculty trust them sufficiently to approach them to discuss any problems or plans. Faculty readily go to administrators to discuss problems of individual students. One professor summarized one facet of trust: "The degree of trust of the dean in the faculty is extremely high and that promotes creativity and productivity of the faculty."

COMMUNICATIONS

Both faculty and students report pleasant surprises and continuing satisfaction with communications in the school. The surprises relate to initial contacts with the school. Written materials were sent to faculty promptly on their expression of interest in applying for a position, and they were impressed with telephone follow-up on the questions they asked. They are most enthusiastic about the interview process:

> The faculty are very sophisticated in their interview approach, which was very impressive; there is a lot of class here.

> The interview process was better than in five other places I went. I was interviewed in a more intelligent manner; and I appreciated the searching questions from a senior faculty member.

> Faculty are carefully selected; all are selected as carefully as I was.

> Faculty come with a clear idea about goals and mission of the school.

> Expectations are clearly spelled out in writing and are pointed out from day one. Goals for the school are delineated annually.

Faculty are confident that they know the channels of communication; they like the fact that communication flows freely across department and hierarchical lines.

Students are impressed by the same facets of communication as the faculty. They received written materials that fully describe the university, the school, and the programs. They comment about never having to wait for answers--from time of first communication with the school, through the application and admission process, and at critical junctures throughout their schooling. They speak of receiving telephone calls in response to questions, but mostly about calls from faculty members expressing the faculty's interest in having them enroll in the school.

"They made me feel that they really wanted me here." Many students remark about receiving answers during the admission period to questions that required several mail communications from the school. Responses to inquiries were individualized letters, not merely forms. Students find that their first impressions about communications persist throughout their tenure in the school:

> From day one, my advisor gave me descriptions of exactly what I would be doing for the whole two years. Now I can get questions answered on the spot. There is great faculty support and advisement at all junctures in the program.

Initial and continuing communications are important to faculty and students; those in the school describe plans and processes of communications as receiving needed attention and working effectively.

STUDENTS ON COMMITTEES

Undergraduate and graduate students have an active part in the administration of the school by means of service on all standing committees. Both faculty and students express pride and satisfaction in the students' participation: "Students have a real contribution to make; they work hard and are listened to." "The faculty listen to us, and they use the input we provide. We are respected for our contributions." Student involvement on committees is another channel for building student-faculty relationships. Students report committee experiences to peers in their student organizations, and faculty share with their peers information and insights about student interest, needs, and abilities. Each group achieves greater knowledge and understanding of the resources possessed by the other. Membership on the school committees moves student organizations to a cohesiveness within the organization and encourages them to think through ideas that can advance the work of the committee for the good of the school. Students respond with excitement on grasping the larger picture of the school's functions and on working on programs that will serve wider needs. Many students say that they try to share their experience with fellow students but are sorry that all students cannot have the active, maturing experiences of committee participation. Student membership on all standing committees is an established component of the administrative organization; it is viewed as mutually beneficial to faculty and students, and, more important, as a resource for enhancing all relationships and programs in the school.

EXCELLENCE

Frequently heard on the campus of a renowned university are expressions of impatience with mediocrity; even more frequently, there are vehement declarations of the need to build toward excellence. There is acknowledgment of high-quality programs and scholarly achievement but never a statement that excellence has been reached. Administrative and academic leaders communicate varied and repeated reminders about the need for movement toward and commitment to excellence. Actions taken to work toward excellence include search for employment of faculty members of the highest quality from throughout the nation; recruitment of high-quality students; curriculum evaluations and modifications; collaboration with scholars in other disciplines; use of outstanding community facilities and institutions for instruction and research; promotion of scholarly research; matching resources to ideas; and associating with scholars throughout the nation and the world in conferences, collaborations, and publications, as well as with visiting lecturers and professors.

The school of nursing contributes to and benefits from the university's support of programs dedicated to excellence. The dean is credited with keeping the faculty and students conscious of a striving for excellence and with a willingness to listen to new ideas and to provide resources for development of new programs. Curriculum goals include development of nurse leaders in practice, teaching, research, and administration. There are high academic standards for student achievement in all programs. Students are frequently reminded about the standards and are helped to meet them.

Some direct quotations convey the feeling about the school's commitment to excellence:

> There is a congruence between goals and what administration supports with resources.

> Makes working here challenging. We really try to build toward excellence.

> There is a vision of excellence that undergirds goals toward which all strive.

> We have identified areas that are futuristic, for example, some graduate programs; we must continue concentration in our thinking and planning to keep in touch with the vision of the future.

> We're never satisfied with what we have; we're constantly reviewing and improving curricula and programs.

> Our goal is to prepare clinically competent individuals. Continually stress to students that their education never ends, requires a continuing professional commitment.

> Mission is excellence in nursing service.

Ours is a whole environment of wanting to be the best.

The university is renewing its commitment to teaching through support of a center for teaching excellence. The center provides a full-week workshop on teaching during the orientation period for all new faculty.

They recruit high-quality students and then help them to be admitted.

Curricula are set up so the school achieves its goals.

It is a pleasure to be excellent--although tiring, it is also stimulating.

Chapter 3

FACULTY

The faculty are extensively credited for the ranking of the school. There are citations of quality and variety equal to those used to describe administration. The influence of the faculty permeates all components of the school's makeup and programs.

EXPERTISE AND DIVERSITY

To the umbrella question, "What makes your school a top-ranked school of nursing?" the most frequent first response was, "The quality of the faculty." This was expressed in several ways, including "competent, hard-working faculty"; "faculty strive for excellence all of the time"; "quality and variety of faculty with different strengths that complement each other"; "faculty gifted, scholarly, dedicated, loyal"; "outstanding, creative faculty"; "faculty are an elite group, very talented and very creative"; "faculty are clinically competent"; "faculty are very well educated and they keep knowledge updated with continuing education." These generalizations were backed up with details about faculty expertise.

Faculty members have extensive and varied educational backgrounds. Some 45 percent hold doctorates that have been earned from universities across the United States. The school makes a practice of a nationwide search for the best available scholar to fill each vacancy. Even though a large number of faculty members are alumni of the university or school of nursing, there is still a variety of expertise; faculty members have degrees in different disciplines, and they have developed expertise in varied knowledge and clinical areas. One faculty member summed it up as follows:

> There is so much expertise in this faculty, if you need to know something, there is someone here who is an expert.

A junior faculty member commented about senior faculty by saying:

> I came here because of the reputation of the faculty. I am constantly impressed by the strong knowledge base in all areas: clinical, theory, health care policies and issues, curriculum, and teaching.

Students contributed:

> Faculty have strengths in different areas. I have not had a course where faculty have not been competent in the area. I am sure part of recruitment is to keep each area strong. Faculty are experts and great resources of information for students; they really know what they are talking about.

Faculty members are viewed as excellent role models in areas of concern to students: clinical practice, teaching, research, interpersonal relations, community involvement. The role modeling is manifested in varied faculty activities: classroom teaching, one-to-one instructional guidance, patient care in the clinical setting, contributions to professional organizations, school and university committee responsibilities, and developing relationships with laypersons and professionals in other disciplines to develop settings for clinical experiences in community agencies.

Essentially, faculty members begin the faculty role with considerable expertise in varied knowledge and performance areas, and they continue to enhance their capabilities in breadth and depth. Their motivations for growth are personal interest and curiosity, and response to interests and needs of students.

Diversity

Characteristics mentioned second only to expertise among faculty members are variety and diversity. There is diversity in clinical focus and in educational and experience backgrounds. There is diversity of research interests and investigations, teaching strategies and theoretical frames of reference, nonteaching activities in the university and the school of nursing, societal and professional issues and activities. There is a mix of faculty: new and old, young and older--"a nice mix." There is an acceptance of diversity among faculty and students; the acceptance is not merely tolerance, but the strengths of individuals are exploited for the enhancement of the learning and production of other individuals, groups, and the school:

> The system supports diversity; not everyone has to be one of the same mold.

> There is an intellectual engagement. Individuality is respected. Each faculty is viewed as a unique individual; shining stars; yet, each can share self and stay unique.

Commitment

Faculty members have their own interests and expertise, yet each is committed to students and to the nursing care of patients. The commitment is shown in their giving of themselves to guide students and provide care for patients. Engagement in these activities would seem to be a full-time task, yet concomitant with those related activities is a persistent drive to learn more, to improve, and to grow in knowledge and competence. Faculty members set high standards for themselves, and surrounding all activities is an aura of concern for improvement--they wish to do things better, to enlarge their knowledge and competence so that their contributions can be greater. The drive for improvement is identifiable in their assigned tasks of teaching and clinical practice and is demonstrated by engagement in continuing education programs and in research. Another focus of commitment is community health care. All, as individuals, are engaged in community activities, and all participate in activities to fulfill the school and university mission to contribute to the improvement of the community's social welfare.

Still another commitment of faculty--individually and as a group--is advancement of the concerns of the profession of nursing. Some faculty members hold elected and appointed positions in state and national organizations of professional nurses. They participate as individuals on their own time, and they serve as representatives of the school in promoting, advancing, and implementing programs of the nursing organizations. At any one time, there are two or more faculty members serving as site visitors for NLN accreditation visits. Faculty members serve as writers of test questions for State Board Tests and engage in two- to three-year assignments on task forces and blue-ribbon committees for development projects of state and national nursing organizations. Faculty members also serve on grant-review committees of the Division of Nursing of the Department of Health and Human Services. Faculty members serve as consultants to education and service agencies in local, regional, national, and international areas. Again, they accept invitations as individuals or as representatives from the school or professional organizations. One faculty member has spent the last eight summers in consultation to the health care services in Indonesia. Essentially, these commitments seem to stem from faculty members' sense of obligation to use their knowledge and capabilities to serve others. Faculty members in top-ranked schools seem to find that the greater their capabilities, the greater the obligation to share them in service to others. "Faculty rise to meet all criteria we have to; yet, most of us are going above and beyond. We overproduce, strive to always give a better performance."

A major component of faculty commitment to improvement of themselves and of the profession is their involvement in research and publication to report and share their thinking and new knowledge. Collaborative groups develop to share ideas and the excitement of investigations. In many instances, the groups yield subgroups that further advance the work. Groups frequently form in relation to the work of a funded project, but funding is not an essential element. There is marked evidence of the value faculty place on publication; they see it as an obligation to society, to their students and school, and to themselves, as well as a means of sharing the results of their efforts.

Research

Besides contributing to growth and learning, engagement in research is viewed as contributing greatly to the quality of teaching. It adds a dimension of interest, immediacy, and excitement to instruction. Faculty who are engaged in research integrate ideas from their own research into their teaching; they also, more frequently than faculty not engaged in research, include the findings and thinking of other researchers in their teaching. Many faculty researchers receive teaching awards. In addition, faculty researchers are apt to be a part of cross-country networks. They are in communication with well-known researchers across the country and they make those persons seem real to the student. They are able to attract other researchers as visitors to the school. An additional impact of the faculty member's research in her teaching is that, almost insidiously, students accumulate a knowledge of the research process and find themselves asking research questions and attempting to design means of discovering answers to their questions. They become aware that the problem-solving process occurs almost automatically as they plan care for their patients.

The permeation of research into teaching and other activities was seldom described in full detail. Rather, it is revealed in discussions of the various activities and responsibilities of faculty members. Consistently, regardless of the focus, some comment would be made about a research-related idea or action.

Flexibility

Another accompaniment of research is change. Next to expertise and diversity, flexibility is an attribute most often ascribed to faculty, and there are detailed descriptions of flexibility of plans and programs designed by faculty members--all of which, of course, is intimately tied to research and the new knowledge it produces. New knowledge is valued because of the base it provides for effecting improvement, and improvement means change. Where research is done, change will be accepted without question, hesitation, or fear. In a top-ranked school of nursing, the early questions asked about change are how best to effect the change, by whom, and when. One never hears the question, "Can it be done?" The collaborative involvement of faculty and students in the research endeavors continues, and the same collaborators move on to plan and implement changes.

It may be presumed that the habits of sharing that develop during research and planning make the resulting change seem like a natural occurrence. The planners and initiators seem almost automatically to provide early information to all who will be involved in effecting the change or will be affected by it. They begin with information and move quickly to involve those to be affected in the planning and implementation of change. It is undoubtedly this facet of effecting change that accounts for the label of "flexibility." Actually, the faculty, through increased knowledge and intensive thinking, propose means to improve the program; they inform those who might benefit from the change; and they invite them to make choices to suit their own needs. They make explicit what is involved in the change and ensure their willingness to implement the changes. The beneficiaries see this as flexibility; the faculty see it as improved program.

It is possible to identify many recent and developing changes effected by faculty: changes in curriculum, clinical practices, teaching strategies, and others. There is movement away from the assignment of faculty to one level of courses and toward most faculty teaching courses for baccalaureate, master's, and doctoral students. Essentially, this is being done on the request of faculty themselves. They see the process as providing for greater interaction among all faculty members and promoting greater opportunity to share and learn from colleagues. They comment about it, particularly in relation to research and clinical practice, which, of course, is another example of their concern for continued learning and improved competence.

The warrant for a top-ranked school of nursing is ascribed to the quality of the faculty: their expertise, diversity, flexibility, and commitment to students, patients, and personal and professional development and contributions. Identification provides only an overview of encompassing attributes of faculty. All can be described more definitively by elaborating the contributions of faculty to the amalgam that is a top-ranked school.

RESPECT, TRUST, COLLABORATION, COMPETITION, COMMUNICATION

Respect for One Another

A balance of stability and novelty marks the faculty structure. New people are integrated into the established cadre of faculty and continuity of structure is maintained. Overall, faculty are mature, work well together, and are very positive toward each other. They maintain a professional colleague-ship, and are open in sharing ideas with others. Mutual respect and trust is pervasive, to the end that faculty have an amazing awareness of the interests, expertise, and program involvement of all fellow faculty members. The aware-ness and willingness to share lead to engagement and extensive support in collaborative projects--curriculum, teaching, research, and community services. Faculty members comment that colleagues are great human beings, people who really care about one another. They report that faculty members support their beliefs in others by commending colleagues and expressing genuine pleasure at another's achievement and success. A special point is made of providing posi-tive feedback for a colleague's program, publication, or award.

A major manifestation of the shared respect among faculty members is the repeated evidence that there is one integrated faculty. Senior faculty plan and implement an extensive orientation for new faculty, including a period during the first year of a one-to-one mentor-learner relationship. The senior faculty members derive satisfaction from being able to contribute to the growth of younger faculty and from the stimulus the arrangement provides for their own continued learning. The junior faculty have only glowing descrip-tions to make of the program: "Senior faculty treat us as peers." "We learn so much--much more than just the layout and program of the school; the senior faculty have such knowledge and are so willing to share." Some faculty members refer to the experience as participation in a buddy system, with all the positive aspects of that concept. Early in their experience at the school, junior faculty develop an awareness of the integrity of the faculty and a confidence in the trustworthiness of their colleagues; when faculty members say they will do something, they follow through on their word. All faculty members have input into many decisions and programs in the school. Input from all is welcome and given thoughtful consideration; from this develops a sense of accomplishment and belonging and awareness of the respect that all faculty have for each other.

Using Knowledge and Strengths of Peers

"Everyone has something to give," and because of the camaraderie and willingness to share, faculty do not hesitate to seek assistance and ideas from colleagues. They not only seek help for themselves, but freely refer others to individual faculty members who possess particular knowledge, interest, and skills. In part because opportunities to pursue personal interests are dependent on the cooperation and planning of peers, faculty members in turn are willing to share their knowledge. Faculty are fast developing into a community of scholars. Faculty members have opportunities to offer and to seek collaboration with peers when developing curricula or when discussion with a peer teaching in particular focus areas on another level might enhance the plans and presentations of both. Other occasions for collaboration are sharing in the many facets of scientific investigations and planning for activities that will contribute to the health care of the community. Such sharing is particularly effective when the contributions derive from learning experiences for students. This makes the experiences more meaningful and alive for students and contributes to the public's understanding of nursing and nursing education. Faculty of the school are viewed by nurses in the community as true professionals; they, as much as colleagues, seek the contributions faculty can make in their particular areas of concern. Faculty provide programs, workshops, and increasingly, consultations; also increasingly, faculty seek collaboration with their colleagues to enlarge and enhance the contributions they make through consultation provided to nursing organizations, hospitals, community health agencies, and other schools of nursing.

When faculty are invited to provide programs or consultations outside the school, they have a heightened awareness of their own expertise; in consequence, they sometimes initiate collaboration with peers. This in turn obviates any hesitance a faculty member might have in seeking assistance from a colleague. It extends as far as inviting colleagues to visit each others' classes and rendering a team teaching situation nonthreatening. There may have been a time when the willingness to share and the temerity to ask occurred only within departments or specialized interest groups, but in a top-ranked school where the faculty are unified, there is no reticence in seeking and sharing ideas, knowledge, and skills.

Constructive Competition

Besides, perhaps because of, the high calibre of faculty, there is a fine spirit of competition, which is a constructive force in the school. Because of the strong feelings of collegiality, awareness and respect for the competence of others, desire to see others grow and succeed, and commitment to the excellence of programs for students, engagement in competition with colleagues is very subtle. Faculty members seek competitive situations for the stimuli they provide; they press forward in their own endeavors in expression of the competitive drive, yet they persist in sharing thinking and resources with colleagues. Their ultimate goal is what is best for the group and for the school; their personal achievement is to that end. Friendly competition is used as it serves to stimulate maximum achievement. Some have suggested that the competition of faculty members is against themselves and not against others. Because of the drive to work together for programs best for the school and for students, faculty members engage in friendly competition, always with full awareness of their competitors. The spirit of cooperation overshadows any negative stresses that might derive from the competition.

Support

A pervasive component of faculty relationships is that of support. There is support among special interest groups, support by senior faculty for junior faculty, support on a one-to-one basis for personal needs and for learning and career development needs. Should a faculty member want to try an idea or a program, there is support on various levels from colleagues, the school, and the university. Should a faculty member be asked to provide a program or contribution outside the school, she need not beg for assistance; rather colleagues will volunteer to cover for teaching and other school responsibilities. Faculty members readily accept invitations to present particular materials in a class of a peer.

Faculty seem to particularly appreciate peer support in evaluations and critiques of material written for publication. They comment that they would not hesitate to seek such critique; they are confident of truthful and supportive feedback. Also, when it comes to planning a new course, faculty members are completely comfortable in seeking assistance, feeling certain of receiving encouragement. Younger faculty come to the school seeking the opportunity to associate with famous faculty members. They soon learn that developing a relationship will be expedited by their famous colleagues, who do not wait for younger faculty to come to them, but rather initiate interactions. The younger faculty members learn that experienced faculty members will listen to them attentively and will give careful consideration to materials with which they seek help. Relationships among faculty may be summed up as superbly cooperative and supportive.

Agreement and Disagreement

The prevailing atmosphere of cooperation and cohesiveness does not preclude disagreement. Faculties must deal with issues, and issue connotes a variety of facts and opinions, without one "right" side. The faculty struggle with an issue openly; they argue, debate, disagree. But the thoughts expressed and statements made consistently focus on the ideas rather than involving individuals or personalities. Faculty members are free to agree or disagree, to express their own thoughts and beliefs; each will be listened to, each expression will be respected. All understand the process and are aware that the ultimate outcome of such discussions and deliberations will be identification of collective goals that will be pursued in a unified way. Faculty feel a freedom to disagree, but they can work together. The faculty dispute openly; cliques do not develop. When an area of disagreement persists after a course of action is decided on, those carrying out the action can move forward with assurance of support for their work--the spirit of collegial disagreement will not interfere with progress. There will be cooperation with a view toward the attainment of excellence in program for students and the total mission of the school.

Communication

Communication among faculty members is extensive and varied. Perhaps the most important result of communication is clarity of all the goals of the school--program, course, class, and student achievement goals. Goals are delineated following extensive exploration and input from all concerned--administration, faculty, students, and consumers. The delineation of goals is accompanied by rationales, plans for attainment, and material for evaluating the degree of attainment. Communication flows freely between department and special interest groups, which in turn maximizes the contribution that each group has to make to the whole. It limits repetition in programs and enhances effective sequencing of program components. In turn, materials are communicated to all who will be involved in and affected by attainment of the goals. Communication is conveyed through many media--verbal, written, graphic, and pictorial. Aside from instructions themselves, faculty communications are essentially planning--planning for new courses and programs and planning for revisions, but always planning for improvement, growth, and excellence. Faculty communication has a purpose; it contributes effectively to the accomplishment of the programs and goals and fulfillment of the school's mission.

CONCERN FOR STUDENTS

Commitment to Students

The faculty's commitment to students is manifested and described in many ways. Some comment that undergraduate faculty members sometimes mother the baccalaureate students, while others say that faculty are very supportive of students without mothering them. Regardless of viewpoint, such comments are always accompanied by examples of faculty members' expressions of concern for students. Faculty are caring and supportive and do everything possible to diminish stress experienced by students. They are fair in dealing with students, make explicit what is expected of them, and provide feedback so that students know at all times how they are doing. In clinical experiences, faculty not only tell a student what she is doing wrong, but take time to recognize things the student is doing well. Their support of students encompasses encouragement and ego building; students are reminded that they are developing into well-qualified professionals and will go on to become leaders in nursing. Frequently, faculty members convey the idea that they simply assume that students will pursue graduate study as part of their career development--alluding, for example, to the time "when 'we' take our PhDs." Commitment is described as faculty members' willingness to "go the extra mile" to assist individuals and groups of students.

Advising Program

Faculty and students report similar views of faculty advising. Faculty members are available to students as needed. The faculty load and low student-faculty ratio allows time for thorough planning with each individual student.

Faculty members are knowledgeable about the programs and help each student select courses to advance the student's own interests. They are able to suggest and plan individualized programs to enhance the student's attainment of goals and to fit the individual's personal needs. Faculty are flexible in planning with the student to facilitate learning; they weigh pros and cons of a student's plan and help the student recognize the best path to follow. Both groups comment about the difference in advising provided in the school of nursing from that provided in other schools in the university. Moreover, students and faculties of other schools comment on the difference in terms of distress, wonder, admiration, and envy. Some students spend up to two years in liberal arts courses before formally enrolling in the school of nursing, yet nursing faculty provide program advising during those years. The quality of advising advances students' programs and contributes to lower attrition from the nursing program.

Viewing Students as Individuals and Adults

Faculty say, "It's a nurturing environment; students are not numbers, they are known individually. They are important to us and they know it." Students say, "Faculty see me in the corridor and call me by name. They treat us like adults, like colleagues from the beginning to the end of the program. Faculty are very sensitive to students as individuals, and they are accepting of different personality types. The students value that they are valued by faculty."

Despite a large student body, students are handled personally. They know that they can go to faculty members with all types of concerns and that they will be listened to and will receive help. Students may have access to any faculty member at any time. They are aware of and respect lines of communication, but there is no rigidity to preclude seeking assistance from any individual faculty member. Faculty members, for the most part, know all other faculty members, their interests, and expertise, and they freely refer a student to colleagues when they might best serve the student. Students view faculty members' expressions of personal interest in them and enthusiasm for their program plans as real bonuses obtained from their experiences in the school. Students find that programs, social events, and special learning experiences are well publicized. In addition, each student has a mailbox, which faculty members frequently use to communicate with individual students. Students remark on the respect and caring on the part of faculty members this demonstrates. They comment also on faculty members' recognition that students have a life outside the school that is important to them. Students see all these things as manifestation of respect for them as individual adults.

Further evidence of faculty members' respect for students as individuals and adults is accounted for in reports of various programs and actions. A student-faculty committee is charged with monitoring and planning to meet the needs of students. It creates a strong bond between students and faculty. According to one individual, faculty members are "entirely dedicated to spending as much time with every student as is required." Besides assisting with students' concerns and planning for progress during their program, faculty members are generous with time and know-how to assist students in looking at job possibilities. Faculty members not only share their knowledge about sources of funding with students, but will intervene on behalf of students seeking funds. Many use students as teaching assistants and research assistants and may even use some baccalaureate students in paid employment on research projects. Faculty members are highly aware of students' personal needs, they are understanding and sympathetic and adjust programs to serve individuals and groups. Some students and junior faculty describe themselves as "amazed" when recounting the evidence of faculty members' respect for students as individuals; none dismisses it as insignificant.

Planning Learning Experiences

Beside extensive planning for curriculum and courses, faculty expand considerable energy and time planning and modifying programs to meet needs and interests of individuals and groups. They are receptive to new ideas and they listen and give serious consideration to proposals that students make for changes. Faculty members do not dismiss their responsibilities with the guidance and instruction of groups of students. They devote time and energy to interacting with individual students with the aim of meeting their individual needs. Individualized learning is a constant focus for faculty. They do not rely on coincidence alone for this; they devise opportunities for interactions with students to promote clinical and didactic learning. These efforts are not lost on students. Surveys and studies consistently report students' appreciation of the learning environment established for them. Faculty members use frequent evaluations and provide students with feedback and counseling as guides to further effort and learning.

Faculty members do the ground work in planning and attaining access to particular clinical settings for groups of students. Beyond that, they provide students with information about each clinical setting and, to the fullest extent possible, make provisions for the student to have experience in the setting of her choice. For graduate students and registered nurse students, arrangements are frequently made for the student to have a clinical experience in a geographically convenient location. In addition to appreciating faculty members' efforts in making special arrangements for individuals, students see this practice as enhancing rapport and collegiality between students and faculty.

Quality Experiences for Students

Faculty members monitor the care provided to patients in the settings where students have clinical experiences. They work with clinical staff to promote the most comprehensive and highest quality care possible with today's knowledge and technology. Should the quality fall below an acceptable level and no improvements be forthcoming, faculty members will withdraw students from the setting. Moreover, on behalf of equity and professional socialization for students, faculty members will refuse to use a clinical agency that wishes to be selective of students. Should an agency choose to exclude some students on the basis of national origin, sex, or race, the faculty would look elsewhere for their students' clinical practice. Faculty members declare a primary concern for instruction and development of students, but of no less importance is their commitment to nursing care for all persons in need of it.

Supporting Students Through Program Completion

Faculty and staff of the university and the school of nursing are student centered. All go to great lengths to support students through the completion of their programs. Students traverse an extensive and discriminating process of selection. Once selected, however, the student becomes an integral part of the school, and extensive effort and planning are expended to assure her progress to a successful conclusion--attainment of her goals. In the school of nursing, the selected student becomes "one of the gang," and the "gang" provides encouragement, reassurance, assistance, and general wherewithall for succeeding. A colleagueship is developed with other students and with faculty; supporting and enduring peer relationships are developed in the student's areas of interest.

One student portrayed the support of the faculty for students' successful completion of program and attainment of goals by describing an episode of hospitalization. Fellow students and--most memorable to her--faculty members visited her and planned ways for her to fulfill her course requirements. She was able to maintain progress and was not delayed in completing her program of study. A graduate student commented, "There have been rough periods, but always there has been support. Faculty listened to me--planned ways to help and ways that I could help myself." Faculty propose that students help other students; on occasion, a faculty member will discuss and encourage a one-to-one arrangement between two students, with offers of support to them. Students frequently note that "everyone really wants you to succeed."

Faculty-Student Socializing

To faculty members, their obligation to students encompasses promotion of growth, development, and socialization in all aspects of human accomplishment. They envision the product of their efforts as individuals who are fully con- tributing members of society and who experience confidence and satisfaction in interacting with others to achieve self-fulfillment. In addition to providing the learning experiences needed to achieve professional nursing status and competence and planning for education in the arts and humanities, the faculty plan opportunities for formal and informal socialization to develop confidence in social interactions. These include formal experiences, such as receptions and award ceremonies; semiformal programs of seminars, distinguished lec- turers, and exchanges of research ideas; and informal brown-bag lunches, picnics, and barbecues. Each type of activity is supported and encouraged by faculty, with sometimes faculty members and other times students assuming the greater responsibility. Promotion of activities may be done by an established student organization or, occasionally, by a group on an impromptu basis. Comments about social events include: "Faculty bend over backwards for students" and "Student organizations in the school are strong, and have some activity in the planning or implementation stage at all times."

Preparing Professionals and Good Nurses

Faculty members are greatly concerned with assisting students to become active professionals and good nurse practitioners. They extend themselves to keep up with things "for the students." They try to keep up not only with the latest in nursing care, but also with the latest in people's lives and living. The school includes in its mission the preparation of professionals who will move throughout the United States; the faculty feel an obligation to know settings and conditions in which the graduates will work.

Faculty serve as mentors to students not only in formal arrangements for courses, but also through example and suggestions about professional responsibility for engaging in research and publishing. Faculty belong to and are active in professional nursing organizations; they pique students' interest by reporting back to them from planning and program meetings in which they have participated. Faculty members use various opportunities for associating with people in other disciplines through engaging in organizational functions as well as in formal instructional arrangements within the school. They have subtle ways of reminding students of the interactions and processes and their meaning for professional behavior. They help students recognize opportunities and ways of presenting a positive image of nursing to the public. One faculty member expressed the depth of her concern for students in saying that she is a teacher because of "the opportunity to influence students to 'love nursing.'" A student recognized the faculty concern in saying, "They work with us; they really want us to become good nurses."

FACULTY REPUTATION AND PRODUCTIVITY

Many factors might be viewed as synonymous with faculty reputation and production, including research, writing, publication, renown, respect, and demand. A major element in the reputation of a school is the quality of the research of the faculty, which is most widely known because of the publications of the faculty; and publications are often viewed as the production of the faculty. In earlier years, faculty members became known through their activities in local, regional, and national nursing organizations. At that time, their writing was generally about administration, patient care, and nursing education. Faculty members and their school continue to become known through these channels, but in the past decade the bulk of publications have included elements of research.

Research and Publications

Most writing and publication of nurses today contain some allusion to research. Some nurses write and publish to share findings from their own research and contribute to the knowledge that is basic to a developing profession. Others write about the research process to assist developing researchers and move more nurses into the mainstream of fully functioning professionals. Nurses writing about the many concerns of nurses also cite research to enhance their explanations and provide credence to their writing. Nursing faculty help prompt nurses to become researchers by including courses on research and statistics in baccalaureate programs.

Faculty members have many opportunities to have their writings published. "Publishers come to the school in droves," commented one individual. The publications for which faculty members contract are most frequently textbooks of scopes ranging from comprehensive coverage of a broad area of nursing care to pamphlet-sized expositions of a discrete technique or teaching strategy. Regardless of the scope of the idea and completed work, the interest, encouragement, and support offered by the publisher may be what finally moves a faculty member to write for publication. Once a faculty member begins writing, she receives extensive empathy and support from administration and faculty colleagues. Essentially, when a faculty member comes to the school, she knows that she will be expected to be productive and that part of the productivity must be in research and publications. Faculty members encounter these activities as soon as they join the faculty. Junior faculty receive encouragement and support from senior faculty. Collaborative arrangements on research projects and even on writing tasks are common devices to promote involvement in these important professional projects. The faculty of a top-ranked school have a major influence on the curriculums of schools of nursing and on the profession of nursing through their textbooks and journal articles.

The influence of nursing faculty is beginning to extend beyond the interests of nursing alone and is having an expanding impact in overall health care and the areas of social welfare and behavioral science. Reports of research done by nurses are being published in journals of other disciplines, and nurses are being recognized as people who can speak with authority in many areas of human concern. Faculty members become known through their writings and are asked to serve on national and international commissions, including president's commissions; planning, review, and policymaking commissions of foundations and federal agencies; and boards of directors of national hospital and medical associations. Nurses are employed as vice-presidents and chief executive officers of hospitals, and as vice-presidents, vice-chancellors, and provosts of universities. These are all positions of influence that go beyond the concerns of the nursing profession but in which nurses have much to contribute. The advancement of nursing into positions of power and influence may be largely attributed to the work, research, thinking, and writing of faculty members in top-ranked schools of nursing.

Research, in addition to being a primary element in the reputation of the school of nursing, earns a reputation for individual researchers, who in turn are known by researchers in other schools. They become known for their track records in securing funding for research and for their competencies in sharing their knowledge and expertise with others through teaching, lectures, and programs, as well as through writings. Faculty researchers attract other scholars and high-quality students to the school. They attract invitations to serve in many ways throughout the country and internationally--one more mechanism through which the school's program is enhanced. The researchers themselves declare that they gain more than they give in the programs they provide away from the school. They bring these gains back to the school to be shared with colleagues and students as their teaching gains depth and breadth; and students are exposed to growing scholarship and to the world around them.

Faculty have been described as indefatigable, "terribly productive" workers--they work during interims, they own computers, they work at home. Faculty members' prevailing interest in and production of research is not lost on students:

> Baccalaureate students have famous researchers as instructors.

> I had heard the names, but I had no idea they were living, walking human beings. It is so impressive to have them as teachers.

Faculty and the University

The national reputation gained by the faculty through their publications have served them and the school in good stead in the university community. Faculty members are known and respected by the faculties of other schools on campus; a cadre of faculty members who are collaborating in research with other faculties is developing. Faculty members are asked to teach classes, and many serve on doctoral committees in other schools; some hold joint appointments. The nursing faculty in a top-ranked school hold power within the university. Nursing faculty members are appointed and elected to major university committees and have access to power within the university. Nurse faculty have been elected to chair such structures as the university graduate studies committee and the university senate. They influence major university decisions and are known in the university as persons who are knowledgeable, caring, and verbal and get the job done. They are perceived as nursing and health care leaders in the community.

Faculty on the National Scene

Many faculty members hold elected and appointed positions in national nursing and health-related organizations. They are members of boards of directors and of special interest commissions and task forces. They are resource people, with excellent communications among peers throughout the United States. They have good connections with faculties in other schools of nursing. Moreover, the involvement of faculty members in national organizations makes major contributions of service to the larger community in many areas of human concern through, for example, the contributions of an expert in theory development in nursing; a member of a national commission on health policy; a consultant in quality assurance to the American Hospital Association; or a pioneer in the application of computer technology to the planning of nursing care in rural communities.

SUPPORT AND ENCOURAGEMENT OF STUDENTS

Adult Learners

A manifestation of faculty members' concern for students as adults merits highlighting. From the day students enter the educational program, faculty members stress that students will be expected and encouraged to be independent learners. Faculty members remind students that they are adults embarking on a career in which they will be expected to assume responsibility for their own continued learning and for their actions in relation to others. Students believe this introduction serves them repeatedly throughout their progress in the degree program; they look back on it as a major influence on their progress toward graduate education. Students suggest that among the elements of this support and encouragement are "pushing" them to engage in new activities such as research and challenging them to try out their own ideas, even at the risk of occasionally being wrong. Faculty members remind students that they are well qualified and that they are going to be leaders in nursing. They help students understand the advocacy role through examples of collaborating with members of other disciplines to plan and implement programs of health care. Through these experiences, students learn to identify the particular aspects of care that nurses can best contribute and the means of being effective in making these contributions. Besides planning efficacious learning experiences, faculty members display a flexibility that allows students to progress along paths of personal interest and at a pace comfortable to the student.

Student-Faculty Peers

As a concomitant to faculty support and encouragement, faculty have a way of conveying to students that they respect them as peers. Graduate students describe this more often than do baccalaureate students, but there are occasions when undergraduates feel it too. The RNs in the baccalaureate program particularly notice and appreciate these relationships with faculty. One RN commented, "I came with a good body of knowledge, and they eased me into recognition that I did have a lot to learn." Faculty members encourage students to seek consultation with other faculty members regarding particular situations of patient care that they encounter during a clinical experience. The idea is to help students develop the habit of going to the experts to enhance their contribution to the care of their patients. Still further evidence of faculty members' respect for students as peers is their encouragement of students' sharing in writing and publication responsibilities. Faculty members have ways--both planned and incidental, overt and subtle--of helping students become aware of the developing peer relationship and confident that they are worthy of the implied respect.

Faculty members do not provide guidance only in the classroom. Students report that faculty members leave messages in their boxes or even call them if they have an idea about something that might be useful in relation to the next day's clinical experience or to a paper or program that a student might be developing.

Support in the Clinical Setting

Of all learning experiences, it is in the clinical setting that students most appreciate support and encouragement from faculty. They comment about on-the-spot supervision. Senior students remark in a tone of wonder about the ready availability of faculty supervision:

I am out there functioning independently; yet, should I need it, the instructor would be there.

It really gives you confidence to try things about which you are sure, but not quite sure.

Some students describe it as a sixth sense; faculty members really understand what being in a clinical setting means to students.

TEACHING STRATEGIES AND CURRICULUM

Creativity in Curriculum

The dynamic faculty members never lack for creative ideas pertinent to curriculum. They state that what they do not think of, students do. Examples of innovations included descriptions of integrating research concepts through-out the curriculum; introduction to computer application in various areas of nursing concerns and provision of hands-on experience and beginning computer literacy in the baccalaureate curriculum; and increasing numbers and variety of clinical experiences in rural and out-of-hospital settings. Each semester's work builds on the previous one, and the faculty devise subtle ways to ease students into increasing complexities, integration of knowledge base, and planning and implementation of nursing care. The faculty are credited with being the most stable element in the school, but the curriculum, one of their largest responsibilities, is the most fluid. It undergoes continuous changes, with major overhauls effected at frequent intervals. The faculty are creative, and much of their creative thinking is focused on curriculum.

Master Teachers

Most faculty are master teachers, with all the competence, strategies, and dedication that description implies. They are well educated and able to communicate their knowledge to others. Yet they know their limitations and make referrals as needed. They set realistic goals and provide students with a total class plan at the beginning of any course. They assign learning experiences as students are ready to handle them so that students develop basic skills before moving on to more complex ones. These faculty members enjoy teaching and receive many awards in recognition of their skills.

Strategies

It is not the purpose of this report to describe teaching strategies, but it is important to note that faculty in a top-ranked school devise and use a large variety of strategies for providing instruction. Examples include use of visiting lecturers and use of personal experiences that provide learning by anecdote. Students view these as effective for their learning; they attribute the apt use of instructors' experiences to the high level of clinical compe-tence on the part of the instructors. The active involvement of students is used extensively in a variety of ways. Of course, students are active in clinical experiences, but there are many other student activities as well, including group projects for community health programs and for class presentations; in-class case presentations; critiques of colleagues' papers or reports; self-evaluation following single clinical experiences and at the end of a clinical sequence; and use of video and computer-assisted learning programs. Many of the strategies are designed to allow self-pacing as well as repetitions and reviews. Undergraduates do not necessarily refer to teaching strategies as such, but they enthusiastically describe various processes that instructors use to provide them with information and opportunities to learn and to develop skills. They credit instructors with making their learning time and endeavors effective.

Students frequently mention examinations as helpful to learning, particularly the feedback that faculty members provide in association with them. The students recognize value in the use of tests made by organizations and commercial testers. They believe that tests patterned after the National Council Licensure Examination (NCLEX) are helpful in preparing them for state board examinations.

In addition to remarking about faculty members' expertise, awareness of student needs, and understanding guidance in clinical experiences, students comment on the learning opportunities provided by nursing service staff. These staff members involve them in care. Students have opportunities to observe staff interacting with patients, and the instructor helps them to evaluate the quality and process of care provided by staff. The students value the variations in care and patient situations that the associations with staff provide. In many clinical experiences designed for senior students, a staff nurse serves as a preceptor over a period of weeks. The students have only praise for this learning opportunity: "It is the real world."

Faculty members who are responsible for particular course content or clinical experiences utilize various teaching-learning configurations. One group might develop a series of learning modules and use criterion-referenced testing as a part of the experience for the students. Faculty members clearly delineate capsule or course objectives; some will then encourage students to try various ways of attaining the learning needed to achieve the objectives. Some groups have developed tutorials, with faculty or other students serving as tutors. For large classes, faculty members develop facets of the teaching to be accomplished through small-group sessions and attempt to have students remain as members of a group with the same one, two, or three faculty members over a prolonged period of time--a full semester or even a full junior year. Faculty members encourage students to submit evaluations and proposals, enhancing students' learning and conserving time and energy.

Thinking: A Process of Learning

Faculty members encourage creativity in students. Students are aware that faculty frequently do not proffer answers, but guide students in ways of finding answers. They help students develop and refine problem-solving behavior. They allow students to be individual, providing a degree of direction, but encouraging students to think through their own versions of meaning and best actions. Students are allowed to fail, confirming the concept that achieving a goal is not always the most important thing in a particular learning experience; rather, learning the process can be of greater value. Faculty members frequently remind students that they will not know everything; of greater concern is that students learn to cope with varied situations, to think them through, and to have confidence in their own judgments.

Emphasis is on independent, critical thinking. There are many opportunities to remind students of the need for and efficacy of the problem solving. For example, the student will learn to use one type of intravenous equipment, but in another setting, equipment will be different. The student must be able to reason through the use of the similar, yet different, equipment. The faculty encourage students to consider various ideas and ways, and then to try one!

FACULTY AS PROFESSIONALS

Faculty commitment to professional organizations is manifested through a variety of involvements in and on behalf of these organizations. Faculty members belong to one or more national nursing organizations and to organizations of other health care or related disciplines, and they are active at the local, regional, and national levels. Activities include holding office, serving with planning and implementation groups, and providing programs for organization meetings. These involvements have the mutually beneficial effects of helping the faculty members to grow in their careers and contributing to the achievement of the mission and goals of the organizations. A further benefit is the visibility such involvement provides for the school and for the profession of nursing both in the community and nationwide.

A major impact of faculty involvement in professional organizations is the role model it provides, which contributes to the socialization of students into the responsible, caring profession that is nursing. Students recognize faculty activities as the fulfillment of responsibilities to the profession and to the society that supports it. They are even more aware of the overt sharing by faculty of their activities and their learning from their various involvements with organization programs. Faculty report to and discuss with students the activities, planning, and decisions evolving from particular organization meetings. They invite students to make suggestions for means of advancing the programs and commitments of the organizations. On the local level, faculty members plan ways to involve students in meetings and activities for community programs.

The number of regional and specialty group organizations of nurses has greatly increased in the last decade. This has led individual faculty members to become affiliated with more organizations and has necessitated difficult choices in setting priorities for allocating time and energy. Essentially, one or more faculty members belong to all major subgroups of the American Nurses' Association, and most of the subgroups with clinical or practice focuses also have faculty members from the school. In recent years, faculty have become more future oriented. Individually and collectively, they keep abreast of what is going on in the profession and in the health care system.

As new concerns or focuses are identified, one or more faculty members assume responsibility for keeping informed and for becoming involved and providing leadership in developments. Their involvement ensures that nursing makes appropriate contributions to policies and programs. Faculty members have become increasingly politically active, with considerable influence on state and national legislatures in development of laws affecting health care delivery and the practice of health care professionals and other workers. The beliefs, actions, and involvement of the faculty publicly portray and define the profession of nursing.

NURSING PRACTICE

Clinical Competence of Faculty

Faculty members are clinically competent and maintain their competence in various ways. Some hold joint appointment with the school and the nursing service of the university or an affiliated hospital; some are employed part-time in a clinical setting; others maintain private practices in the community. A primary path to keeping current in knowledge and skills is through clinical instruction and supervision of students, which includes sharing the planning of patient care with students and staff in the clinical setting. Still another way is through direct contributions to care of patients as a part of a consultant role. Faculty members also engage in consultations at agencies not used for student experiences. They conduct clinical research and apply theory to patient care as well as assisting students and staff in refining their skills in theory application and identifying research questions. Faculty members are well respected in all clinical settings in which they are active, and students see their own recruitment for employment by the hospitals in which they have experience as a sign of respect for and confidence in their instructors. Faculty are obviously committed to a high quality of care for patients and to the guidance of students in becoming skilled nurse practitioners and conscientious, caring professionals.

Focus on Clinical Practice

From its inception, a primary concern of the school has been health care of people. This concern is conspicuous in the curricula of all programs in the school, in learning experiences provided for students, and in community service projects of the faculty and students. From their first nursing course, students are provided with opportunities to contribute to the health care of people. Nursing interventions and provision of care for patients are integral parts of all nursing courses, from the introductory nursing course for undergraduates to the clinical courses required of all doctoral students. The majority of research done by graduate students is investigation of questions formulated during care and observations of patients. The school, faculty, and students are committed to high-quality nursing care in all clinical care settings. Moreover, students find the clinical courses of such interest that many take one or more clinical courses after they graduate.

Access to Clinical Care Settings

Faculty and students have access to many and varied settings for clinical learning experiences and for research. Nursing faculty enjoy a colleagueship with faculties in the schools of medicine, pharmacy, public health, and others, leading to increased sharing of courses and exchange of faculty for classroom instruction. The faculty also have peer relationships with nursing administration and staff in health care agencies in the community. In recent years there has been positive accomplishment in bringing together people in nursing education and nursing service. There are joint appointment arrangements for faculty and staff, and the increase in numbers of clinical nurse specialists and nurse practitioners give considerable impetus to the development of ties. The use of staff nurses as preceptors for senior student clinical practicums has involved even more agency staff in close association with school faculty and allowed input from practicing staff nurses into the educational experiences of developing nurses.

Faculty members seek sites for optimal learning experiences for students. Although these are mainly found in relative proximity to the school, including the university hospital, faculty may be involved with clinical agencies over a wide geographic area since using more distant agencies is convenient for students who may live far from the school. Making arrangements for student clinical learning experiences is time-consuming and detailed. Faculty must interact with many individuals to secure permissions and cooperation and to formulate schedules. Lack of availability or access to a sufficient number of patient care settings frequently adds to the chore of providing clinical settings for student practice, but faculty of a top-ranked school do not experience this difficulty. Many more agencies extend invitations for students to use their facilities than there are students who need to use them.

Besides the care that students provide the patients, there are many benefits to an agency in having students. A large benefit is the stimulus students provide staff to strive for a high quality of care. Staff also benefit from learning opportunities in interacting with students and faculty, sharing in some student case conferences, and consulting with faculty. For many, interaction with students provides an impetus to go on with their own formal education.

Another link between the faculty and the nurses in clinical facilities is effected through planning meetings. Administration and staff of one agency invite faculty and key staff from the various agencies used by the school to a late summer meeting. Information is shared and student experiences in the agencies planned for the coming year. In the spring, the same individuals are invited to the school for discussion of the past year's experiences. Staff from the agencies report their experiences with students and faculty and make proposals for changes that might enhance the situation for staff and the education of the students. These two meetings permit staff and faculty to get to know each other and allow necessary communication about the shared experiences as well as individual and mutual responsibilities for the care of patients and education of students.

Providing and maintaining access to quality clinical facilities for student learning experiences and research is a complex endeavor requiring cooperation among large numbers of people with varied responsibilities. Comprehensive planning and open lines of communication can make it work to the benefit of both the student receivers and the agency providers. The faculty deftly maintain relationships that provide broad benefits to the students, the agencies and staffs, the school, the patients, and the community.

FACULTY EXPECTATIONS OF STUDENTS

Scholarship

Faculty have set high standards of scholarship in all areas of study: liberal arts, support courses, and nursing courses. A top-ranked school is not an easy school; there is concentration on critical thinking, analysis and synthesis, and application of theory in the real world. Expectations are clearly delineated for students and reinforced through feedback that allows students to know about their status and achievement throughout the program. Students are fully aware of what the faculty expect in the way of scholarly work and writing. Faculty members encourage involvement of students in research activities, which they use to enhance their awareness of scholarly behavior and results. Students are repeatedly challenged to think beyond what they currently think; they are pushed to creativity and innovation. The school provides a demanding, intellectually oriented environment.

Independence and Responsibility

Faculty members communicate expectations to students about development of initiative, independence, and accountability. They set high standards to serve as the basis for development of personal responsibility. They help students recognize the many responsibilities of a professional person to self, colleagues, patients, employer, community, and society. Faculty teach students to be responsible for their own learning and encourage them to support their classmates in collaborative and competitive ways in the achievement of learning goals. They use experiences designed to increase independence and responsibility to help students develop a conscientiousness about their own behavior and a spirit of caring for patients and fellow human beings. They use self-evaluations, evaluations of courses, and critiques of nursing care provided by others to help students acquire sensitivity and awareness of conscientious, ethical behavior. Accountability is concomitant with independence and responsibility. The functioning and goals that are evidences of these attributes are inextricably mingled, yet students must become aware of the nuances of each. Faculty members support their expectations of students developing into responsible, professional nurses by guiding them toward awareness and experiences that call for the exercise of professional behaviors. They help students understand that professional behaviors stem from and are manifestations of personal feelings and motivations of independence, responsibility, and accountability.

Developing Professionals

Faculty expect students to be involved in more than mere attendance in the classroom or clinical setting. They expect them to engage in activities that are expected of a professional person: belonging to organizations, attending meetings, and becoming involved in organizational activities designed to advance the goals of the organization and provide services to the community. Faculty members provide ideas, support, and encouragement to students in these activities. They remind students that they are developing professionals and leaders and that both roles imply initiative, engagement, and dedication to advancement of the profession, extension of its knowledge base, and improvement of its practice.

COMMITMENT AND RESPONSIBILITY

Faculty display a dedication and commitment to the many and varied aspects of their responsibilities. They are loyal to the school and to their responsibility for the education of students. They are committed to a high quality of nursing care and to the improvement of the care. Faculty members will do what needs to be done for the school or for student programs, even when a task may not be their primary choice.

The faculty perceive themselves as continuing learners and are committed to scholarly pursuits in various forms, including formal course work, attendance at organizational meetings, familiarity with current literature, and informal discussions with faculty and student peers. They have high expectations for themselves; they feel obliged to improve. They see themselves as responsible not only for their own improvement, but for contributing to the improvement of the profession and of nursing practice. Some faculty members suggest that their school is on the cutting edge of progress in nursing, and there is only one way for them to go--forward. They are committed to excellence in nursing practice, education, and research. The faculty express complete confidence in their status and abilities as leaders, and their thoughts and plans are to continue to lead. They are a major factor in the top-ranking of the school, and they intend to maintain that status.

Chapter 4

STUDENTS

For universities and schools, the reason for being is students. Focus on students is essential to rationalize the need for and describe the many people, facilities, and other resources that make up a school as well as their inter-relationships; yet, in most of the descriptions, students are only a tacit focus. Despite focus on students being fundamental to descriptions of all other elements composing a school, only a few specific descriptions of students are needed to describe their particular concerns and involvement.

QUALITY OF STUDENTS

Outstanding Students

The students in all groups--baccalaureate, master's, and doctoral--are of very high quality and come with solid educational backgrounds. Most students in the graduate programs enter with good clinical backgrounds and well-defined goals. Because some 20 percent of BSN students hold degrees in other areas, and others are RNs, many baccalaureate-level students also have delineated goals to which they are committed. Students are attracted by the caliber of the school; it takes a certain motivation for students to choose to enroll in a top-ranked school. They are committed to themselves, their program, and the school, and they work very hard. The depth of preparation is an asset to the school and to fellow students. Students bring a wealth of experience to seminars; they provide continuing challenges and stimulation to faculty. Students in the doctoral program are bright and knowledgeable; they contribute to the quality of the instruction and programs of the school--informally, through social exchanges and classroom and clinical participation, and formally, through assistantships and consultations to students, faculty, and community health agencies.

Standards for Admission

The school has high admission standards for all programs. Selection criteria are spelled out and adhered to. If students are expected to complete the program successfully, they must come well prepared. Students appreciate the high standards and view themselves as "the cream of the crop." They say that the knowledge and abilities of fellow students and the interest and expectations of faculty stimulate them to work at their own highest potential.

Student Pool

There is a large pool from which to select students. In the pool for each degree program are students from across the United States, with the doctoral program having the largest number from areas outside the state and region.

Each program has scores more fully qualified applicants than can be accommodated. Moreover, all pools of potential students, including that of baccalaureate students, continue to grow. Faculties of other schools ask that rejected applicants be referred to them, knowing that most will be well qualified for their programs. In each of the past two or three years, there have been some 500 percent more fully qualified applicants than could be accommodated in each program. This allows a very high caliber of student to be selected and a good mix of student to be admitted. The latter is particularly important for certain graduate programs, where association with competent individuals who have common interests can greatly enhance the program for all students.

LEARNING: SELF-MOTIVATION AND INDEPENDENCE

Self-Motivation

Although there are variations among individual students and those in different degree programs, that students are self-motivated is a well-warranted generalization. Many have been employed and returned to school to work toward defined goals; their motivation for studying and learning is very high. Students come to programs expecting rigorous demands on time and energy; for the most part, they don't fuss about it. Conversely, as one faculty member put it, "Our students have high-level grumbles: 'I don't have time to learn everything I need to know.'" Self-motivated students are apt to have firm ideas about what they want to learn. Their motivation and goals are encouraged and supported by faculty, but faculty members also challenge and direct them into areas of study required for their programs. The students are aware that learning is not merely memorizing and completing an assignment. They know that they are expected to increase their thinking abilities and pursue learning about a subject beyond the confines of the assignment described in the course syllabus. Students know that they are free to seek assistance from faculty, to ask questions in class, and to suggest associations among related areas of knowledge. Students in the baccalaureate program follow their own motivation in using the learning laboratories; those in graduate programs rely on libraries and computer or research centers to pursue study as their self-motivation dictates.

Independence

Self-motivated learners are apt to display considerable independence in their pursuit of learning. This behavior is fostered by the faculty in various ways: through continually enlarging and updating materials in learning laboratories and in libraries; reminding students of resources for independent study and practice; assisting, or providing assistance for students as they use the study resources; and including course assignments that require independent study. Courses designed for independent study are of high quality; they demand more of the student than the classroom format and students respond positively to the demands.

Students are encouraged to take responsibility for their own learning. In response to students' questions, faculty members frequently provide guides to sources of information or to processes for solving problems, rather than immediately supplying an answer. Students gain a sense of professionalism through becoming involved in their own learning. For example, students design and implement various community health service and teaching projects. They see themselves as making a difference in health care for particular groups in the community. As students assume more and more responsibility for independent study, they make a growing commitment to continuing their learning along both informal and formal paths.

Early in their programs, baccalaureate students are guided in learning the process of obtaining knowledge from various sources. Graduate students are assisted with refreshing their skills. Both groups are assisted in identifying what is important for them at any particular time or in relation to particular problems. They are reminded and encouraged to build on their own backgrounds of knowledge and experience.

CONFIDENCE

Students have very positive self-concepts. They are confident of their abilities to learn and to perform. Their confidence has many sources. They have experienced success in previous educational endeavors, and they were selected from among many bright, qualified applicants for admission into the school's program. The faculty are a primary source of students' confidence; they reassure, respect, and encourage students in various learning achievements. Faculty members foster creativity and provide students with freedom to pursue individual interests and paths to achievement. Students are aware of their own developing knowledge and skills; they can cite evidence of the ability to apply the knowledge and use the skills competently. Staff in clinical agencies comment to students about their abilities and performance, and they report their approval to the students' instructors. Students see themselves as developing professionals, and graduating seniors declare that they are capable and ready to care for patients in many settings. They are proud to be nurses.

DIVERSITY

There is great diversity in the total student body; the mix of characteristics exists in each degree program and parallels that of the student body of the university. There are differences in educational, socioeconomic, ethnic, and work experience backgrounds; national and international places of origin and current home; educational goals; and professional interests. There is a wide range of ages, with an older median age for baccalaureate students than in the majority of baccalaureate programs in the United States. Increasing numbers of baccalaureate students are part-time students, mothers, and holders of degrees in other disciplines.

One registered nurse student described the meaning and value of the diversity as follows:

> We have a wide range of cultural groups. I am becoming aware of biases I had; I associate with "outsiders" and I recall what I once thought; I ask, "Was that me?" We really get to know other life-styles and ways of thinking; we become aware that others may have better ways than our own. We learn not only from students in the school, but from those in other schools on campus.

Faculty find the diversity a challenge; students in all degree programs find it exciting and a true asset to their total educational experience.

RESPECT

Students and graduates merit and receive respect. Agencies invite faculty members to bring students to them for clinical practice, and they seek graduates for employment on their staffs. The school prepares baccalaureate students for real clinical responsibility, and graduate are prepared with clinical expertise to assume responsibilities in one or more functional roles. Students are capable of making choices of where they should function. The graduates are fully prepared for the next level of formal education.

Nurses are coordinators of all patient care and are leaders in planning and implementing programs for long-term care. All graduates are aware of professional responsibilities and have ideas about activities in which they will engage to fulfill them. Increasingly, students and graduates are involved in politics and policymaking. The school's graduates gain regional and national reputations through achievements in nursing and other health care actions and through publications, some of which were done while they were still students. They are respected not only by other nurses, but by consumers and members of other professions as well. They are sought for membership in community, state, and national health care planning groups. Their reputations are reflected in attitudes of respect for the school, the students, and the graduates.

STUDENT ORGANIZATIONS

There are established and activie baccalaureate and graduate student organizations in the school. Students become members of their respective organization when they enroll in the program. Many become involved in the activities of the organization through serving as officers and on committees, as well as through participation in various programs. Students are expected to belong to their respective state and national professional student organizations. They attend annual state and national conventions, and some students are usually involved in the meeting's promotion and programs.

Students represent their organizations on various committees in the school and in the university. They are fully participating members with vote on such committees as curriculum, faculty teaching awards, research, and space. The school supports the organizations with student-elected faculty sponsors and with budgets for such necessities as printing and mailing. Each organization has assigned office space. Leaders in student organizations frequently go on to be leaders in state and national professional organizations. Faculty and students view participation in student organizations as a path to educational socialization into a fully functioning professional person.

SATISFACTION WITH PROGRAM

Students frequently express satisfaction with their program; there are few, if any, reports of dissatisfaction. They mention receiving a well-rounded education and being well prepared for nursing. They know that some 95 percent of graduates pass state board examinations. Students are convinced that they have much to offer in their roles as professional nurses. They believe they are prepared for the wave of the future in nursing in relation to the requirement of baccalaureate preparation for professional nurses. The seniors enthusiastically describe the clinical practicum in which they have extensive clinical experience in association with a preceptor. During the experience they are allowed increasing responsibility for care to a group of patients. They develop confidence in their readiness to assume the responsibilities of a staff position in various patient care settings.

Graduate students cite as a highlight of the program development of competence in and the habit of critical thinking. They have a good grounding in research and theory development capabilities. They feel "the school has done for us what it sets out to do." They are confident of being able to do things they want to do as their career develops. They are comfortable about knowing what to do and how to do it.

Students discuss the programs in the school enthusiastically and repeatedly comment about their excellence, with an outstanding component being the collegial relationships between faculty and students. They declare that they are happy to have a degree from their school.

COOPERATION AND COMPETITION

Cooperation among students is frequently discussed. Competition is mentioned less often and always with comments about it being "healthy" in nature. Faculty members describe competition as challenging and stimulating to growth. They encourage it within these bounds, and they are alert to assure that there is also a healthy mix of cooperation. Students express surprise at the limited amount of competition, in contrast to the cooperation and sharing among students. They identify numerous occasions of cooperation. Students are familiar with the experience, areas of knowledge, and backgrounds of many of their peers, and they draw from each other. They are willing to share knowledge and to assist individuals and groups in study, planning, and making decisions about work at hand and short- and long-term planning. Because of their background, cooperation might be expected to occur more frequently among graduate students. However, increasing numbers of older persons are enrolled in the baccalaureate program--for example both a 52-year-old licensed practical nurse, mother of seven, and a 48-year-old retired military officer, father of two, are students in the baccalaureate program. Other students find them to be valuable resources, and "elders" in turn enjoy supporting their "peers."

Throughout the programs, subgroups of students form to share study experiences related to various components of the program. A strong identity and loyalty develops among members of a group, but the groups also manifest a fluidity as students move on to other facets of their program and become members of other subgroups. The experiences of sharing and caring are valuable developmental experiences for students in all degree programs. Faculty members support and encourage such behavior. They are reminders of the cooperation necessary among nurses in providing 24-hour care for patients and as members of multidisciplinary health provider teams responsible for care of individual patients and families and for health care programs for groups and communities. Students have many and varied opportunities for sharing, and they seem fully aware of the value of these experiences for developing habits and strategies of cooperation.

Chapter 5

CURRICULUM

In the university and the school of nursing, there is a vision of
excellence that becomes the goal toward which all strive.

--Administrator, Boston University School
of Nursing

EXCELLENCE AND QUALITY OF PROGRAMS

A major hallmark of the school is the excellence and quality of its
programs. The school has a long history of academic and clinical excellence
in all programs. This excellence is expressed through rigor of course work
and commitment to very high standards. Faculty believe that program quality
begins with their commitment to excellence in education, both clinical and
academic. The results of paying close attention to curriculum are the strong
programs that emerge. Faculty members describe their continuous involvement
in curriculum development and revision: "We continually look for ways to
upgrade curriculum. We evaluate continually. We try to keep up with what is
going on out here; then accommodate needed changes into curriculum."

Faculty believe that attention to curriculum pays off in strong academic
programs that attract quality students. The pool of applicants to the various
programs is large, even in a period of generally declining enrollments.
Faculty characterize students as self-motivated and independent, adding that
students have to be independent, since the environment is not structured.

Graduate students appreciate their education. They state that the
curriculum attracts a lot of students who can meet the rigors of the program
and produces knowledgeable graduates. They know that everything they will
learn will improve the quality of their practice. They describe the depth of
the core courses and related cognate courses in their programs, noting in
particular that required core courses give good preparation for entering
specialities at the master's level. The doctoral core courses highlight
nursing science, leadership, research, and theory development. Courses at
both levels fit together into a whole to produce a neat, finished product.
Graduate students view the flexibility that faculty have built into the
graduate curriculum as important: "It allows us to develop areas of personal
interest while simultaneously preparing in declared majors."

Undergraduate students say a great deal about the excellence of their
program of study. They particularly like the way the faculty have organized
the courses in the nursing major. A number of their statements reflect this
appreciation:

Classes are well organized, reading material is suited to courses.
Courses are well delivered, with good lectures.

The way the program is set up is excellent; really prepared for each level you go to.

Skills are learned on a 1:1 basis. Really decreases anxiety because you know you've done it.

Each semester builds on the previous one and faculty ease us into increasingly complex stuff.

Fairly structured beginning of the program but changes to less external structure. There's increased flexibility in the senior year, that becomes self-guided learning. This promotes more personalized learning.

The junior year needs to be highly structured. There's a weaning process--works very well and it's well-timed.

Nice progression of courses that guides you along. . . . Also good integration of courses at any one time. They all relate with each other.

Students remark that the prerequisite courses are heavy, but give a well-rounded background, providing a good university education. They believe the liberal arts and sciences foundation gives a sound basis that prepares them well for practice. It prepares them to look holistically at clients to whom they give care and to view the psychosocial as well as the physical.

Undergraduate students believe that reasoning is well taught, and they see this skill as important to the practice of nursing. They think that the faculty have a balanced view of the clinical and the theoretical. They believe that the courses offered and the clinical experiences in the curriculum make theirs an outstanding program and that it is a step ahead of many other schools.

Students believe that their education has prepared them to be autonomous professionals and that making changes is within their power. To them, professionalism connotes responsibility, and the education and knowledge that they gain in their program equips them to assume responsibilities for changing health care and the image of nursing.

The high quality of the educational programs in the school results from the collective contributions of faculty, students, and administrators. Faculty members commit themselves to the development and revision of curricula to keep them timely and responsive to current societal needs. They take their responsibilities as teachers very seriously, preparing well for them and sharing their individual and collective knowledge and expertise with their students. Students assume their respective roles as independent, motivated learners. They understand clearly that quality programs of study are rigorous and demand a great deal of work on their part. They work hard to measure up to faculty expectations and to take full advantage of the many learning opportunities available to them in the university, the school, and the clinical settings. Administrators work hard to provide a productive learning environment within the school. They offer the guidance, support, and resources needed by faculty and students to maintain and enhance the high-quality programs in the school.

AUTONOMY

Faculty have a great deal of independence and autonomy in carrying out the responsibilities of their role in the school. They have control over curriculum policymaking and view this as an important strength. Since the various curriculums are in a state of continuous evolution, faculty control provides authority to make needed changes. Yet, the accompanying responsibility ensures that changes will maintain the high quality and integrity of the curriculum. The authority of faculty members with regard to curriculum change is not exercised lightly. As one stated:

> The faculty is the most powerful group in the school. Their freedom to decide the direction of curriculum can influence the direction of the school. . . . There is a good sense of power in the faculty, and they take responsibility for their work, for shaping their environment.

Autonomy is also accorded to students. Students in all programs exercise autonomy in designing programs of study to achieve their own goals. They draw up personal goals and objectives, arrange their own clinical placements in agencies of their choice, and assume increasing control over their own learning. Along with increased self-direction, students experience freedom to develop their own ideas, especially conceptual frameworks for nursing practice.

BACCALAUREATE PROGRAM

Five major elements characterize the baccalaureate program:

-- A variety of options for building individual student programs.

-- A clear structure with an internal flexibility.

-- The concept of preparing a generalist.

-- A strong clinical component.

-- An integrated curriculum with several major processes emphasized, including critical thinking, independent nursing judgment, professionalism, the application of theory to practice, and nursing research.

Variety of Options for Building Individual Programs

During the past decade, the student population seeking admission to the baccalaureate program has changed dramatically, as adults returned to or began school after pursuing other interests and goals. These "new" students make up about one-third of the student body and have needs that are different from those of earlier student groups. In response to these needs, faculty have developed various options to help students achieve educational goals. Now considered an integral part of the program, the options take the form of acceleration and deceleration (i.e., pacing) of the course of study. As faculty describe the option:

> The intent is to allow people to use their time wisely. It allows for individual interests. It doesn't penalize students for illness or deceleration. . . . It's the disciplined, organized, motivated student who accomplishes the same objectives in a shorter time.

A cross section of students take advantage of the options: traditional (18-to-22 year-old), full-time students; older students; students with previous college degrees; part-time students; and students with registered nurse or practical nurse backgrounds. Although different names are applied to the options, they all take into account students' previous educational and life experiences. The faculty treat students as adult learners who possess different needs, and they work hard to help students expand their previous knowledge bases. For students with previous degrees, faculty work to mesh the knowledge they possess with the new nursing knowledge. For students who are unable to attend school full-time because of work or family responsibilities, classes may be organized in a number of ways: late in the day or in the evenings; concentrated into one day rather than spread across a week; on weekends; or at extension sites closer to students' homes. The goal is to provide a variety of ways for students to meet educational goals--to make education available to them.

Faculty members believe that students benefit from the variety of options available to them:

> All of this diversity prepares students to cope well in the real world. There is no one way; students must make conscious choices among alternatives.

> Students are highly motivated, independent adults, who do not need a structured environment to learn.

Faculty members view their own role as that of:

> Challenging and guiding students into appropriate areas; students are not forced into one mold.

> Working with students to establish the students' goals.

> Facilitating student learning; weighing the pros and cons of students' plans and helping them determine the best path for them.

Students realize their own diversity and comment on the faculty's comfort with expanding their previous knowledge base. Their appreciation of the variety of options open to them can be seen in one student's statement:

Openness and flexibility are refreshing in a world of gatekeepers.
Can design one's own program; I can sit down and discuss my program
goals with faculty; there's no rigidity.

Clear Structure with Internal Flexibility

Although there is less flexibility within the baccalaureate curriculum
structure than in either the master's or doctoral programs in nursing,
opportunities for flexibility do exist. These commonly take three forms. The
first is the opportunity to obtain the baccalaureate in a variety of ways as
just discussed. The second is the elective course option, a traditional part
of baccalaureate education. What is distinct in the top-ranked school of
nursing is the increasing number and variety of nursing electives available
for students. The electives are offered during the summer sessions as well as
during the traditional fall and spring semesters. Some electives are solely
classroom courses, but the major portion have a practice or clinical component. Through such offerings, usually three to six required hours in the
upper-division sequence, students have an opportunity to develop greater
knowledge and skills in an area of personal preference, and faculty members
have an opportunity to teach in areas of personal interest.

The third area of flexibility is the large variety of sites and agencies
available to students for clinical experiences. Using guidelines developed by
faculty in line with the curriculum objectives for the level or course,
students are able to exercise choice in the selection of particular sites for
their clinical experiences. Such flexibility enables some students to arrange
clinical experiences in settings closer to where they live. This cuts down on
travel to and from the sites, which is particularly important for students who
have roles and responsibilities in addition to their education. Other students
can gain experience in large, urban health care settings during one semester
and then move to smaller, suburban ones the next semester. Still other
students can choose clinical experiences in agencies where they might like to
work after graduation. Faculty and students value the number and variety of
agencies available for clinical experiences and view this as important in
preparing for the first professional nursing position following graduation.

General Preparation

Both faculty and students are very clear that the major goal of the
baccalaureate program is to prepare a beginning generalist practitioner.
Faculty believe:

We do a good job preparing entry-level practitioners.

Students develop the skills needed to perform as first-level
practitioners.

Students graduate with a great base for beginning practice.

The baccalaureate curriculum is designed to help students prepare to practice as a generalist. Students learn how to use the nursing process with many types of clients and have a great deal of contact in their clinical experiences with clients who have diverse needs. These experiences help students become self-directed. Faculty members attempt to cultivate personal preferences in students, so that by the time they graduate they have a pretty good idea of what they want. The variety of clinical experiences that make up the generalist preparation facilitates this goal.

Students have similar things to say about the goal of baccalaureate education. They believe that the baccalaureate curriculum:

> Teaches you to be a generalist. Shows that we are more than technicians.

> Produces a well-rounded generalist who can work in any situation. Makes us cognizant of self-needs and other's needs. We have a sense of self.

Strong Clinical Component

To achieve the goal of preparing students to practice nursing as generalists, a strong clinical component is needed at all levels of the curriculum. The strong clinical component in the program is respected by employers, who are very pleased with the graduates. Even though the faculty place emphasis on clinical experiences, theory is also stressed, especially the application of theory to practice. The nursing process is used as the organizer through which theory is applied in clinical practice.

During the early part of the nursing student's education, clinical experiences are more structured and have strong faculty guidance. Supervised practice in the school's learning skills laboratory is a major learning process during this period. As students move through the senior year, less structure and faculty presence are apparent. Students assume greater autonomy in choosing the focus of their clinical learning, using course objectives as their guidelines. The autonomy may take several forms: development of each week's clinical objectives and selection of patients or clients that may help meet the objectives; development of contracts or agreements for preceptor-study experiences; or choosing of types of clinical experiences or particular clinical setting in which to work. The last two experiences usually take place in the last semester of the senior year and may occupy from 7 to 15 weeks of the semester.

Students appreciate the structure that surrounds the early clinical experiences as well as its decrease as they move through the program. The statments of several students illustrate this:

> Structure is increasingly appreciated; it increases skills in time management. Organization becomes internalized by graduation. Very clear parameters of what is expected for courses; it puts the responsibility on me.

The curriculum facilitates the independence of students.

Our graduating with BSNs. . . makes us marketable. I'd rather be that than any other type of RN, and we are prepared to assume that role. We can handle anything in general nursing.

Integrated Curriculum

The faculty are very proud of the completely integrated baccalaureate curriculum, in which threads are integrated progressively, including the individual, family, and community as well as all age groups. The courses in the nursing major are highly organized and structured so as to incorporate concepts, theories, and processes with planned clinical experiences. Each course in the program is designed to provide a firm underpinning for subsequent courses. The well-defined integration in the curriculum provides for clear articulation of courses wth each other. Faculty members see this as the basis for quality baccalaureate curriculum sequences. Students are pleased that the coordination of courses and clinical experiences are so very well done. As one noted, "There must be good communication among faculty to achieve this."

Five major processes are emphasized in the baccalaureate curriculum: critical thinking, independent nursing judgment, professionalism, the application of theory to practice, and nursing research.

Critical Thinking. Baccalaureate students themselves are the most articulate spokespersons about the critical thinking process:

Teaches you how to reason; very important to the practicce of nursing.

Makes you think of "whys," not just the "how-tos."

Makes you think for yourself--make decisions; really makes you accountable for your actions.

The curriculum really stresses seeing relationships among things; I really see relationships now.

One student beautifully summarized the students' view in the following statement:

They teach us that we won't know everything. Teach us how to cope with new situations by thinking things through. Maybe it's a mixture of concepts and processes--I'm not sure.

Faculty members comment that critical thinking is stressed throughout all courses in the nursing seuqence, and as a result, students become really analytical. Use of a conceptual approach, not just facts, increases students' ability to analyze. Critical thinking ability is essential in the practice of professional nursing.

Independent Nursing Judgment. In the baccalaureate curriculum, independent nursing judgment is viewed as an analogue to critical thinking and professional accountability. Critical thinking is a prerequisite to professional judgment, which is related to accountability for one's actions. Students realize that they must be safe, responsible, generalist, professional nurses. Their program is designed to provide them with varied opportunities to practice independent thinking, which is the basis for making sound professional nursing judgments.

Professionalism. Developing professionalism begins with students having a strong liberal arts base. This base, gained in the first two years of college, instills a sense of professional self and values in students. "The goal is to give them the groundwork to give them a good start in their careers." Students have many opportunities to learn those components that make them professional from other departments and schools in the university as well as from the school of nursing. The well-rounded program that students receive helps them to look holistically at the clients to whom they give care. Students clearly summarize their understanding of profesionalism in the following statements:

> Curriculum promotes professional development. There's an emphasis on holistic approach in all BSN courses. Stresses the psychosocial aspects as well as the physical. Emphasis is on promoting a higher level of wellness.

> Professional orientation always and an emphasis on raising standards of the nursing profession.

> Mission is to teach professionalism, autonomy, that change is within our reach, and we can change the image of nursing. More rooted in being a professional, and that carries with it a lot of responsibility.

> BSN fosters personal and professional growth as a nurse and as a person.

> Curriculum facilitates students' independence.

Both faculty and students believe that developing professionalism is an extremely important process in the baccalaureate curriculum. Students believe that they develop as professional, not technicians; their baccalaureate program fosters true professionalism, not quasi professionalism.

Application of Theory to Practice. The nursing process, with its focus on the holistic nature of the client, whether an individual, family, or community, is utilized as the integrator for applying nursing theory to practice situations. As a result of the heavy emphasis on the various steps of the nursing process early in the program, students begin to see relationships between theory and practice. Then, with the help of faculty, they begin to use a conceptual approach to analyze why things happen to clients. The knowledege gained in prerequisite courses, such as anatomy, physiology, and microbiology, becomes integrated and used in the clinical settings. Students state that it is like turning on lights. As students progress through the program, their growing integration of knowledge gained from nursing and other disciplines is seen in the types of care they plan and give to clients. Their confidence develops as they begin to see more clearly the relationship of various theories to specific practice situations.

Nursing Research. Both faculty and administration view nursing research as an essential part of the baccalaureate curriculum. They stress that students should be taught to be wise consumers of research, that they should have exposure to becoming readers of research. Students state:

> The research course is a highlight; helps us read research and appreciate it.

> Have a required course in nursing research and it's really good.

> Placed toward the end of the program, research course helps turn on lights.

> The course is taught by good teachers of research, who take us through the whole of the research process, and use their own or other faculty's research as examples to teach us the process.

The undergraduate nursing research course is usually one semester in length, and occurs either in the last semester of the junior year or during the first semester of the senior year. Introductory statistics is required as a prerequisite or co-requisite course.

MASTER'S PROGRAM

Administrators and faculty state that the goal of the master's program is twofold: first, to prepare professional nuses to be specialists in advanced clinical practice, teachers in schools of nursing, and administrators in health care delivery systems, with a strong knowledge base in theory, research, and clinical practice; and second, to provide a foundation for doctoral study. A major concern is meeting the diverse needs of graduate students, many of whom are attending school part-time and working to pay for their education, changing their career goals, and planning to continue on to doctoral study. Four elements can be identified as characterizing the master's program of study: a tripartite curriculum, a variety of curricular options; emphasis on theory, research, and the clinical setting; and expert teaching faculty.

Tripartite Curriculum

The curriculum is structured to achieve the goals of master's study. It consists of three areas of study: a required set of core courses, which all students take early in their program of study; clinical concentration courses; and functional role practicum courses. In the core course sequence, students develop their knowledge base in nursing theory, research, role theory, health care policy and politics, ethics, and leadership. The remaining sequences build on this knowledge base.

The clinical concentration courses are a blend of instruction in theory and selected clinical experiences. As one administrator concisely put it, "Students do concentrated work in an area of interest. It they're in rehab., they can focus on cardiac, or on neuro." A faculty member added: "We have a very clinically oriented program. Role modeling is very important. Faculty's expertise in clinical practice flows into teaching. We never ask our students to do anything we do not do."

The third portion of the student's program is functional role preparation. A practicum experience is designed to give students a number of opportunities to function in the role of teacher, administrator, or clinical specialist under the guidance of agency preceptors as well as faculty. Both faculty and students find the experience particularly valuable. From a faculty perspective, there is a real integration of theory and clinical. Students find that they can use the knowledge gained in course work and perform at a high professional level. They develop confidence that helps them make progress in master's study. Students judge the role focus to be particularly good. They value the field placements because they permit integration in the real world of the various roles discussed in class. They believe that the guided experiences not only encourage their independence but also develop their leadership skills and more advanced professional behavior.

Curriculum Options

The master's program is very flexible and offers students a large number of options from which to choose. The faculty designed the program with flexibility in mind because they believe that graduate education should foster individualized programs of study. They also find that the number and variety of course options give faculty members the opportunity to teach in their areas of special expertise, develop new areas of study as needs arise, and discontinue old areas as needs diminish.

When students begin master's study, they select from the various options available in the program the courses and learning experiences they wish to pursue. Once the required core courses are completed, students again choose more courses and learning experiences from within the speciality concentration and functional role sequences. As one graduate student commented: "The MS program is really flexible; it's flexible enough to do your own thing. Has many options." In other words, the individualized program is the norm rather than the exception in the master's program.

Theory, Research and Clinical Emphases

Faculty teaching in the master's program place strong emphasis on theory, research, and clinical practice, as illustrated by the following comments:

Our concern is about research. We build in more supportive courses on research to give more guidance.

Goal of the master's program is advanced clinical practice.

Nursing research is very strong in the master's program even though thesis is optional.

Clinical expertise at master's level; prepares students to do research.

Strong clinical emphasis in master's program.

Theory permeates the whole curriculum. Students use theory as a basis for all presentations; for clinical practice.

Theory-based practicum courses; MS is very theoretically based.

From the beginning of graduate study, students engage in an in-depth exploration of a variety of nursing and other theories. They are expected to analyze and critique theories and use them as a basis for clinical practice. The research focus includes in-depth understanding of all components of the research process, research criticism, and the development of a research proposal. Students who elect to do the thesis proceed to carry out the proposed study. A faculty sponsor guides the students in conducting the study. Some type of oral presentation before other faculty members and students marks the completion of the process. Students find the thesis option a great learning experience. In particular, they enjoy working closely with their faculty supervisors and other faculty committee members on a one-to-one basis. Students find that the individualized research experience accounts for a great deal of excellent learning.

The master's program is so designed that all students, regardless of functional role choice, receive in-depth preparation in their chosen clinical area. The concentration courses have clinical components, varying in amount depending on the course and the clinical major of the students. All practicum experiences are theory and research based. As one faculty member states: "The goal is to prepare students to understand theory-based research to improve nursing practice." Both faculty and students view the clinical focus as a highlight of master's study:

It takes place in diverse places with all types of clients; develops clinical expertise.

It's great asset in finding jobs after graduation.

Expert Faculty

Administrators describe the faculty who teach master's students as experts with highly developed areas of expertise. They believe strongly that graduate students need exposure to such faculty experts and to a diversity of expertise. As stated by one administrator: "The best faculty teach in this program." The senior faculty, many of whom teach graduate courses, use a variety of teaching methods to meet student needs. A great deal of time and energy goes into their teaching preparation. In addition to helping students to become knowledgeable, competent nurse practitioners, their goals are to develop students' analytic and leadership abilities; to make them aware of current issues affecting nursing and health care; and to keep them abreast of changing societal needs.

Currently, faculty are studying ways that the master's and doctoral programs could be meshed: "We are looking at reconceptualizing the graduate program as a postbaccalaureate undertaking. Some students may exit at the master's level; others could go through to the doctorate."

Beginning evidence of changes is the inclusion of master's and doctoral students in some of the courses common to both levels. These courses have the same requirements and expectations of the students, regardless of the individual's degree goal. Faculty believe that each group of students will benefit from the other's strengths and that the design permits a more holistic approach to graduate education.

Students have excellent access to faculty. Strong collegial and mentoring relationships develop. Graduate students appreciate being treated as colleagues and being involved in ongoing faculty projects. Faculty manifest this colleagueship by asking students for feedback about their personal research endeavors. Graduate students respond very positively to this type of collaboration: "I was so flattered that I was asked to critique their research. I spent hours on it, typed it up, and gave it back to them within a week. I learned so much doing this."

Some master's students serve as research assistants to faculty. Some are employed part-time on grant projects, while others participate as part of course requirements or through independent studies. These types of arrangements help students understand the principles of the research process as well as its application in the real world.

In summary, administrators and faculty state that the master's program is one of high quality and depth of preparation. They believe that their graduates are well prepared to function as leaders in the nursing and health care community and that they make a definite social contribution. Graduate students echo their sentiments:

> The master's program gives you a good basis for the future; it encourages a professional rather than technical outlook.

> There is depth in the graduate program, both in the required core and the elective courses.

> The courses further develop your critical thinking skills.

> The core teaches you about the politics of health.

> Field experiences permit good integration of roles we will play in the real world. It encourages independence and leadership.

DOCTORAL PROGRAM

The goal of the doctoral program is to prepare nurse scholars and researchers who are committed to the advancement of the scientific knowledge base of the profession. This program, which is approximately 60 semester hours in length, is also characterized by definitive elements, some of which are similar to those found in the master's program. The elements identified are a required core sequence of courses; a variety of curriculum options; expert faculty; highly motivated and qualified students; high expectations; strong faculty-student relationships; and resources for the conduct of research.

Required Core Courses Sequence

The doctoral program is organized around a set of core courses. The courses are designed primarily to enhance skill in theory development and testing of theory, research design, research methods, the principles of norm-referenced and criterion-referenced measurement, nursing and health-related issues, and health care policy and politics. Faculty consider that the core provides the foundation upon which the remainder of doctoral course work builds. The following comments by faculty and students illustrate the focus found in the doctoral program:

> Doctoral program is very strong in research, statistics. Measurement also very strong; it runs throughout program.

> Doctoral program has a consistent thrust on theory development. Students develop a theory model for their own dissertations.

> Doctoral program prepares competence in theory development.

> Nursing research is very strong in the preparation of doctoral students.

> Strength of the doctoral curriculum is that there is a core set of courses.

> Students become very knowledgeable in research and politics.

> Structure of doctoral program is farsighted; health policy is very strong.

> Balance between theory and research in the doctoral program.

> A well-developed doctoral program with a strong research program sequence.

> Doctoral program emphasizes theory and research; also strong in health policy.

> Doctoral curriculum designed to develop scholars and leaders in the nursing profession. Great strength in core courses.

Both faculty and students believe that this focus in the core courses provides a solid foundation for professional life following award of the doctorate.

Variety of Curriculum Options

A variety of curriculum options and the opportunity for students to individualize their programs of study is also found in the doctoral program. Students characteristically choose a specialized area of focus consisting of a series of courses which become progressively more in-depth as students move through the sequence. Through the cognate and elective course work, students further expand their knowledge base and become more fully a part of interdisciplinary and interinstitutional academic life. Interdisciplinary collaboration is also fostered through students' dissertation research. Each student's dissertation committee consists of one or more members from other disciplines. For many students, this is their first opportunity to engage in such activity.

Expert Faculty

Faculty members teaching in the doctoral program are firmly committed to the advancement of nursing knowledge through research and through theory development and testing. They are excellent role models for doctoral students who came to the program to learn the skills needed to pursue such a commitment. Faculty are actively engaged in a variety of scholarly activities, including nursing research; grant writing; publishing; consulting on regional, national, and international levels; public speaking; and various types of clinical practice. An expanded account of faculty productivity is provided in Chapter 3.

Faculty members have a great variety of expertise to share with students, who can always find someone to assist them in a particular area of need. Faculty report that a large amount of their time is spent working with students, either one to one or in small groups. The faculty believe that this personalized approach provides the best type of learning for doctoral students.

Highly Motivated and Qualified Students

Faculty enjoy the challenge of working with doctoral students, whom they describe as intelligent, motivated, creative, and committed to the pursuit of scholarship. Students in the doctoral program come from all over the United States and other countries. They value highly the research and theory emphases of the program and the expert preparation of the faculty who teach them. Intelligent and highly motivated to succeed, students describe faculty as challenging, facilitating, catalyzing, and guiding them in their pursuit of learning. Students are eager to learn about theory and advanced research methods and design. They place significant value on their relationships with faculty and with peers, and believe these relationships are a hallmark of doctoral study.

High Expectations

Faculty have high expectations of themselves and of their students in the doctoral program. The curriculum is described as rigorous and demanding. Doctoral students are expected not only to master the elements of theory development, research design, methodologies, but also to apply these principles in their dissertation work. The faculty believe that students must develop their knowledge base in depth and breadth in order to become scholars and leaders who possess the skills needed to advance nursing as a profession. Faculty and students acknowledge these high expectations with pride as the following comments show:

> Nursing research based on theory is strong in doctoral program. We demand rigor. We want our students to stand up to scrutiny. This means good dissertations; and we have some.

> I'm pleased with the depth and scope of course work. I came to doctoral program to learn how to be a researcher, and didn't expect it would be easy.

> Doctoral program is very competitive, but competition is very positive, not harmful. I think it benefits profession because it makes us hardy scholars.

Strong Faculty-Student Relationships

The development of strong relationships between faculty and students is an important part of doctoral study for both groups. Faculty treat students as colleagues from the very start of their programs of study. Although faculty and students share ideas in the usual formal classroom manner, a great deal of sharing occurs on a more informal basis. A variety of mechanisms are used to foster the development of strong faculty-student relationships, including research emphasis groups, which bring faculty and students together on a regular basis to discuss what is happening in a particular field of interest; monthly research colloquia or sandwich seminars, where faculty and students present and critique each other's work; and social gatherings such as picnics, tennis tournaments, and coffee hours. All of these activities provide an atmosphere wherein lively interchange between students and faculty can and does occur. Within such settings, students are socialized not only to the academic life, but also to the role of scholar within the academic community.

Students also place high value on their interactions with each other which occur formally through the graduate students' nursing organization. This group promotes networking among graduate students themselves, between students and faculty, and with professional colleagues in the nursing world outside the university. Doctoral students appreciate having a formal group with which to identify, and view this group as the vehicle that brings them together in times of celebration and in times of need.

Resources for the Conduct of Research

Although Chapter 6 is devoted to the resources of the school of nursing the university, particular mention needs to be made of resources that faculty and students have available to them for the development and implementation of full-scale research projects. In addition to the members of their dissertation committees, doctoral students have access to consultants who are experts in statistical methods, research design, psychometrics, and whatever else they require in order to do their research. These consultants are found in the school of nursing, in other departments, and in the various centers, departments, institutes, and foundations within the university. Faculty and students take full advantage of the rich resources available to them.

In summary, doctoral education promotes the development and refinement of scholarly inquiry in faculty and students. Both groups are committed to advancing the knowledge base of the nursing profession through theory development and refinement and the conduct of research. The combination of the various elements of the doctoral program in interaction with each other provide the essential ingredients for developing the future leaders of the nursing profession.

THEORY

Faculty and students make frequent reference to nursing theory and its role in the three degree curricula. Statements fall into the following three categories: practical application of theory to clinical practice, the relationship between theory and research, and theory for its own sake. A statement from a baccalaureate student reflects the emphasis on theory:

> We use theory all of the time. Roy, Rogers, Orem. We use it in classes and in clinical. Required to use theory in every assignment and paper. Exposed to a lot of theory. We never do anything without it.

Practical Application of Theory to Practice

The relationship of theory and its application to nursing practice is stressed by the faculty teaching in all programs. Faculty expect that students be able to apply theory in the real world and work very hard to help students integrate theory into practice at all levels in the curriculum. Faculty members state that nursing is an independent art and science and believe that this independence is a key ingredient for developing a strong theoretical base for nursing practice. At the baccalaureate level, the theoretical base of practice is more narrow, focusing on a single conceptual framework. In contrast, master's students develop a broader theory base and select their own nursing model to guide their practice. Students' comments depict the focus on theory:

> We never do anything in clinical without a theoretical rationale. Our actions are guided by theory--it gives legitimacy to our practice.

Gives us a solid background in theory as a basis for practice.

Ability to apply theory is emphasized.

Relationship of Theory and Research

Faculty members comment on the balance between theory and research that becomes particularly evident at the doctoral level:

There's a theoretical emphasis at all levels, but it's most outstanding at the doctoral level. There, research and theory are tied together.

Theory is strongly emphasized here, and the main purpose of research is to expand and clarify the theoretical basis for nursing practice.

Students' comments reflect a similar emphasis.

Both theory and research give us a good basis for the future.

Focus is on theory development and research; we look at science in a broader perspective.

Strong emphasis on theory and research.

Theory for Its Own Sake

An appreciation of nursing theory in and of itself is also important to faculty and students. At the doctoral level, faculty and students work with what is the nature of nursing knowledge and what are appropriate foci of study. The goal is mastery of the principles of theory development and critique of nursing theories. Students are conversant with different theoretical perspectives arising from different philosophic positions and develop the ability to justify the stance they take in relation to nursing. At the master's level, students are exposed to a wide variety of nursing theories and encouraged to choose among them those that they prefer to use as a basis for their own professional practice. At the baccalaureate level, students state that there is a strong theoretical basis underpinning all of the nursing courses, and they are constantly referring back to theory. Students view this emphasis on nursing theory as providing them with a strong professional base, as the following two comments clearly show:

We have a theory background. Know why you do what you do and why things are happening to a client. I've never known that kind of critical thinking. I've studied hard. I'm current on theory; technical skills you have to know about, but I think theory, giving reasons for why you do things, is extremely important.

We have an appreciation of theory; it's not just the doing. We think creatively and use the knowledge base.

CLINICAL PRACTICE

All programs of study have a strong clinical focus. Clinical competence of students is the goal. Courses at each level are designed to prepare clinically competent practitioners. Through these experiences, students get a broad picture of the role of the nurse as a member of a multidisciplinary team in a variety of urban and rural health care settings. The following statements from faculty members illustrate the strong clinical components of the school's programs:

> Components within all programs focus on clinical competence.

> Clinical courses are strong at all levels. Good variety of clinical experiences.

> Clinical experience is a strength. Students name it as a strength. Emphasis is on clinical decision making.

Students make similar comments:

> Curriculum is really good for clinical practice. We have the necessary courses to help us in clinical practice.

> Program is clinically focused. Happy with this. I've seen creative applications of the expanded role.

> Clinical placements are exceptional. Qualified people in agencies.

Faculty and agency preceptors give students in clinical settings a great deal of supervision. They encourage students' individuality and originality in clinical practice and do not confine them to practice in traditional roles. Close professional relationships develop among students, their clinical faculty, and their agency preceptors. Students particularly enjoy these individualized learning experiences, stating that this helps them really learn how to function in the professional world of nursing. Students also learn that they "don't end their education at graduation. Lifelong professional growth is encouraged." Everything they learn in their programs of study is of some value to them.

EVALUATION

Although evaluation of programs has always been a part of the school of nursing, it has become a more systematic and formalized process in recent years. Administration and faculty have developed a detailed plan of evaluation that includes the following components:

1. The area to be evaluated.

2. The criteria for evaluation.

3. The people responsible for conducting the evaluation.

4. The types of data needed.

5. The groups from which these data will be collected.

6. The time frame within which it will be undertaken.

7. What will be done with the results of the evaluation.

Administrators and faculty place strong emphasis on systematic evaluation of each curriculum. Faculty members expect that their courses and their teaching will be evaluated regularly. Every course is reviewed on a yearly basis by the appropriate curriculum committee. Those courses that are not taught every semester are reviewed each time that they are offered. Materials reviewed consist of the faculty's evaluation of the course they have taught as well as students' assessment of the course. The clinical agencies utilized for student experiences are also evaluated by faculty, students, and selected agency representatives. The resultant data are reviewed by faculty in order to improve the courses and clinical placements for the enhancement of student learning.

Faculty members look upon the ongoing evaluation of programs as a strength. As one stated: "We're never satisfied with curriculum. Always in process; that's a strength." Students also see the value of ongoing evaluation of their programs and appreciate the fact that their input is valued and utilized:

Faculty are always asking us to evaluate something and see how it can be improved.

They are really into self-evaluation here.

Openness of faculty to criticism; willing to take suggestion from students. Ask for evaluations of lectures, not just at end of semesters.

We have extensive evaluations of courses and they [faculty] take it seriously.

Computerized evaluation is truly utilized and used as a tool in promotions, tenure. We get feedback.

They listen to what we say. When we do evaluations, I feel like they are used to make changes.

They want input from students and want students on faculty committees.

The formalized evaluation process is an integral part of the functioning of the school. All groups (administrators, faculty, students, and agency representatives) participate to some degree in various aspects of the evaluative process. The results of evaluation are valued and used to bring about changes designed to improve the education provided to students. The benefits of evaluation are seen by all involved with the school. The overall desire of faculty to continually evaluate what they do is a key element that "pays off in strong academic programs that attract quality students."

OUTREACH

Administrators and faculty in the school are committed to serving a variety of populations "that need to upgrade their education." The following statement by an administrator succinctly depicts this commitment:

> We respond to the needs of the community to provide nursing education. There's a shared commitment with the community to provide higher education for nurses. And that commitment gets expanded to the state, nation, and world.

Two mechanisms are used to provide educational opportunities to the community: continuing education (CE) offerings and formal outreach programs of degree credit courses.

Continuing Education

There is a department of continuing education in the school staffed by individuals whose primary responsibility is the development of formal continuing education programs for nurses with a wide variety of needs and interests. Administrators and faculty members strongly support the programs through their active involvement as teachers and participants. Administrators view the continuing education offerings as a major vehicle for making positive inroads into the nursing community of their region, their state, nationally and internationally. As one noted:

> Through CE programs, we co-sponsor conferences with organizations. We also contract with state agencies to provide their CE days. We have research days and faculty development days each year and invite the agency community to attend them free of charge. We even have a contract to provide continuing education to nurses in another country.

The faculty believe that the offering of a variety of quality CE programs has made the public very aware of the school of nursing and promotes the school's contribution and involvement with the larger nursing community. Students benefit from the CE offerings. They are invited to attend programs at a reduced rate or free of charge when the programs are for faculty development. Graduate students may be invited to served as CE faculty and present workshops in their areas of expertise. This involvement in CE is an added enrichment to their programs of study and provides another avenue for their service to the community. Faculty and staff in the CE department make a valuable contribution to the education of the nursing community.

Formal Outreach Programs of Study

Formal outreach programs at off-campus sites have been developed and implemented to meet the educational needs of nurses wishing to pursue bachelor's and master's degrees. The programs are located some distance away from the parent campus. Faculty from the parent campus as well as faculty employed at the off-site campus teach courses in the programs. The standards for faculty employment, promotion, and tenure are the same for all faculty, regardless of where they teach. Students also have the same admission criteria and are of a similar caliber to students who attend school on the main campus. Clinical facilities used by students in off-campus paograms are comparable to those used by students attending the main campus.

Despite the geographic separation of the campuses, faculty from the regional campus serve on school and university committees. Telecommunications are increasingly being utilized to facilitate the exchange of faculty members between campuses as well as to share the expertise of faculty with students in all programs. Administrators and faculty members make numerous statements about the value of off-campus programs:

> Outreach programs in another part of the state have made a significant impact in the number of graduates produced there.

> Regional programs make a significant contribution to preparation of profesional nurses in these regions.

> Will offer programs anywhere in the world. We are a university without boundaries; we offer programs where needed.

> Faculty take programs to the communities where students are. We provide service to a population that need to upgrade their education.

> Regionalization is a real strength to school.

A positive outcome of the off-campus experiences for faculty involved in their development, implementation, and evaluation is that they have learned how "to design low-cost, quality programs." This skill has not gone unnoticed by the dean of the school, who has now asked faculty to study the feasibility of extending the doctoral program, in whole or in part, to areas of need beyond the main campus.

In summary, the two outreach mechanisms of the school, continuing education offerings and off-campus formal programs of study, have brought the outside world much closer to the school of nursing and extended the boundaries of the school to encompass the world. As one faculty member so aptly stated:

> These ventures have exposed the school of nursing people to other people in the state and in other countries. We go where there is need. This has increased visibility not only for the school but for the university. Has enhanced our public relations.

CHAPTER 6

RESOURCES

A wide variety of elements in both the university community and the larger community are described as resources available to the school. These range from geographic location, to buildings, to financial support, to information sources; and faculty and students are themselves identified as being resources. Along with excellent administrators, scholarly, interested faculty, and high-quality students, resources are viewed as indispensable to creating and maintaining outstanding educational programs.

LOCATION

Geographic Area

Although top-ranked schools of nursing are dispersed throughout the United States, geographic location, encompassing weather, life-style, and recreational opportunities is frequently mentioned as an attraction for both students and faculty. Some like warm weather, others opt for the temperate, four-seasons climate; some want to ski, others want to sail. Most acknowledge that teaching and studying do not allow as much time for indulging in these pleasures as they would like, but there is satisfaction in knowing that they are there. In general, the school's geographic area is described as one in which people would choose to live. It can be credited as a major factor in the selection of a school for a significant number of faculty and students.

City

The city in which the school is located is credited as a major resource for students and faculty alike. Both groups mention the same attributes as being important to them: the pervasive educational milieu of the city, along with its history of pioneering in education at all levels, and the regional and national renown of the various educational institutions, universities, colleges, and particular units within the larger institutions. The city has cultural centers and programs that provide opportunities for enjoyment, participation, and study in music, the arts, history, and science. A large part of the enriching facilities are the people of many ethnic groups and individuals of world renown. Many are in residence, and others are brought in for appearances of various duration. Facilities and scholars attract other scholars. The city and its atmosphere of culture and education provide stimulating and exciting opportunities to associate with intellectuals and to add to one's awareness and fulfillment.

A close second to the educational and cultural assets of the city are the number and variety of health care facilities, along with schools for various health care professionals. There are medical centers of various size and excellence in many specialty areas, each with national and even international renown. Most important, these facilities have so evolved in the scope and qualities of their programs that the staff members engage in active collaboration with those in every other facility in the city. An individual may practice, study, or do research in one school or center and have complete access to all resources of any other facility in the city and its environs. For the most part, access is formalized through established consortiums or in written agreements.

The city is the state capital or the largest city in the state, a factor that establishes it as the center of resources and power in the state and explains its attraction for intellectuals. Funding sources are there, along with legislative power and influence. In addition, opportunities exist for jobs of great variety, either part-time or full-time. The city that hosts a top-ranked school of nursing is a place where things are happening and where opportunities exist to share in making them happen.

CLINICAL FACILITIES

Number, Variety, Excellence

Clinical facilities are the resources faculty and students alike must be most concerned with and most critical of. Because the school is part of a great university, many resources for teaching and learning may be presumed to be available. For a professional school, it is necessary to ensure that facilities, programs, and experts are available to provide the instructional, laboratory settings for student learning experiences. Fortunately, for a top-ranked school of nursing, extensive clinical resources are available and accessible, including the university hospital and clinics and numerous hospitals, nursing homes, clinics, and community health care agencies where students and faculty are welcome. The school has extensive and varied linkages, both formal and informal, with people and institutions in the community and surrounding region.

Specialty units within the various health care centers excel in research and care for people with diverse health problems. It would be difficult to identify a health condition within the community for which there is no provision for care and study. One faculty member described the community and region as a "microcosm of the United States," encompassing all possible health care situations, with all being available for experiences to students of the school. Mention was also made of the harshness of life in parts of the city, the need for innovations in rural settings, and the opportunities for association with people from various ethnic groups. Experiences in all of these situations are broadening for students.

The professional staff of various disciplines welcome the students. Many of the nurses employed in the agencies, from staff nurses to clinical specialists to directors, are alumni of the school. They are interested in and supportive of the students. Many serve as preceptors to students, who describe them as understanding and caring. Students report that any hospital is available to them and that they have experiences in the best hospital in the community; indeed, students do have experiences in one or more magnet hospitals.

Experts

Nationally and regionally known experts in all specialties of nursing are employed in various settings within the community. Students have opportunities to study them during clinical experiences, and many are employed by the school for particular classes, for continuing education, and for consultations in curriculum and research.

LIBRARY

Students and faculty have access to extensive, varied, superb libraries. The main library of the parent university is outstanding in size, coverage, currency, historical collection, and convenience of access. There are varied specialty collections throughout the campus and at satellite sites. Faculty and students in all schools have access to all libraries, including law and highly specialized collections. Various schools and departments within schools have small, specialized reference collections that also are available to all university scholars. In the school of nursing, departments maintain fairly extensive specialty reference shelves of materials with a five-year limit of currency. The university budget has annual provision for the main library and for library acquisitions by each school.

Besides the book collections belonging to the university, the surrounding community boasts many library resources, including the main library of the city and libraries of professional organizations, industries, other colleges and universities, hospitals, and health care agencies. The university is part of a formal consortium, with agreements that scholars of one institution have access to libraries of any of the other institutions. One student commented, "Any book or document you could possibly need can be found in this city." Specialty libraries develop literature updates each month and they will send copies to anyone on their mailing lists. Indexes of major journals are readily available, and scholars can obtain reprints of articles within a week of request.

All libraries have well-qualified staff. A librarian in the main university library is assigned responsibility for working with a liaison faculty member to update and maintain availability of materials needed by nursing students. This librarian is sensitive and alert to nursing needs; her interest and cooperation are manifested in frequent suggestions for innovations and pertinent acquisitions to the nursing collection. A full-time librarian on the school of nursing staff assists students in locating materials and maintains stock, arrangements, and catalogs of all reference and audiovisual materials in the school of nursing's holdings. Scholars are increasingly availing themselves of computer searches, and there are librarians to assist with these searches and with acquisition of the materials needed for study, whether they be housed in the main library, on campus, in other libraries in the city, or even out of town. Computer use for finding and accessing the literature is free for students, and there are designated funds to assist with payments for other scholars. Thus, nurse scholars have an extensive foundation and support in their library resources.

UNIVERSITY

The nursing school enjoys equality with all other schools in the university. Faculty and students are peers of those in other schools; they are respected as members of the university community and for themselves as individual scholars. They have access to the various programs, classes, facilities and laboratories; sports and recreation equipment and areas; theatre, music, arts, and museum exhibits; visiting lecturers; and special learning, counseling, testing, and health care programs and facilities. Nursing students receive treatment equal to that of students in other schools for scholarship and loan funds; the faculty receive university award and research funds. The university is a total community of scholars who address almost all areas of human knowledge, and contains facilities, equipment, and people to advance and transmit that knowledge. Nursing scholars are an integral part of that community and may avail themselves of all its resources.

The university of which the school of nursing is a part is situated in the cultural center of the state, and enjoys the largest financial support of any tax-supported institution of higher education in the state. The university is renowned in the region and the nation. It is known as a center for research and for the scholars in residence, including one or more Nobel prize winners. It has several departments or schools among the top 20 in various national rankings of schools and colleges.

Both faculty and students comment about "the campus itself" as a meaningful resource of the university. It is a place of natural and planned physical beauty; cluster arrangements of buildings enhance association and make use of various facilities convenient. Obviously, planning has enhanced the total college experience and promoted the largest possible involvement of the students.

Regardless of its exact location on campus or in relation to other structures and facilities, faculty and students comment that the school is optimally situated. They recognize advantages of the location, and none proposes a more advantageous site.

A major source of the university's excellence is the people: the scholars and the people of varied ethnic and national groups represented among both faculty and students. Nursing students are exposed to this rich resource not only in their own school, but as they participate in classes and programs of other schools in the university. Moreover, faculty and staff are aware that the purpose of the university and of their being there is to serve students, to provide for them maximum learning and growing experiences. Equipment, learning tools, and physical facilities are provided, and the people assist students to derive maximum benefit from them. Students comment about the availability of the many assets in the university and about the interest and helpfulness of all people with whom they interact. No matter whom they ask, they are listened to and receive a helpful response.

COMMUNITY

Clinical Resources

The community that surrounds and supports a renowned university encompasses many and varied resources that are assets for the university and for the students and faculty of its many schools. Of primary concern to the school of nursing are clinical facilities; where there is a renowned university there are collaborative relationships with most community agencies, and this is conspicuous in the associations of the faculty and students of the school of nursing with the staffs of the many community health service agencies. Staff members of agencies welcome students and are active in providing learning experiences for them. Essentially, more facilities are available than can be used by the school of nursing; its students are given preference for places over students from other schools. In some of the highly sought clinical settings, nursing students have opportunities to share planning and care with students from other health care disciplines and experience realistic team work. In addition to providing for association and collaboration in patient care with counterparts in other disciplines, these settings usually serve people of various ethnic, and socioeconomic backgrounds, which further enriches the experience.

Other Educational Institutions

Numerous other institutions of higher education exist in the community of the large university: universities, colleges, and specialty institutes. These institutions have formal and informal arrangements for sharing expertise, programs, resources, and facilities. All enlarge the resources available to scholars in the school of nursing.

Other Interests

As intellectuals, faculty and students have interests outside the school and their profession. They find facilities for input and outlet for these interests in the community. For many, the resources in the community are of utmost importance to themselves and to their families. They participate in community activities both as consumers and as providers. They become active in organizations, in school activities with their children, and in recreational opportunities. Resources in the community provide means for full, satisfying living.

Funding and Advisory Committee

Historically, universities have engaged in various fund-raising programs; indeed, they have development offices whose charge is raising funds from various private sources. It is only recently that deans of schools of nursing have promoted programs of fund-raising beyond encouraging their alumni associations to raise funds for student scholarships or for purchase of special furnishings or equipment for the school. Today, the dean of a top-ranked school of nursing has a systematic plan and pattern to promote fund-raising actions. Alumni are still a valued resource. The dean works collaboratively with the university development office, which has assigned a staff member to promote programs and make contacts calculated to interest potential donors in the school of nursing.

In recent years, these efforts have yielded hundreds of thousands of dollars that are being used to endow professorships, support visiting lecturers, provide scholarships and loans for students, and provide equipment or particular teaching-learning projects in the school.

Employment

Opportunity for full- and part-time employment is another community resource of importance to faculty students. Sometimes the decision to come to the school is influenced most by the availability of employment for a spouse. Another significant factor is opportunities for employment following graduation. Students who find the geographic location and all community assets highly desirable during their school experience want to continue to live in that atmosphere.

A community is a multifaceted entity; a community that possesses a renowned university has many resources directly and indirectly related to the university. The total complex of interrelated and interacting factors makes for an enriched educational experience. The university enhances the community; the community makes a great university possible.

LEARNING CENTER

Skills Laboratory

Regardless of the name given to the school's learning resources center, it is extensive, well-stocked, and well-staffed. Its meaning to students can be gleaned from some of their comments:

> You can go back and review techniques. It's a safe place to come back to. Always someone to assist and show how it's really done.

> Almost like a sanctuary--a safe place to review skills, techniques.

> You get your assignment the day before. If I need to do suctioning, I can run downstairs and in five minutes get practice and guidance too.

> Lab has everything you need to do before going into clinical.

> My home away from home. Everything I need is here and I can come and spend the day. Staff know exactly what I need.

The teachers there make it an enjoyable experience.

I can be independent, yet there is help available. The people who have set up the Learning Resources Lab really care about us.

The laboratory has all supplies and equipment that students will encounter in the hospital. In addition, there are textbooks for reference during the practice periods. The center stocks an extensive up-to-date library of journal reprints, textbooks, audiovisual equipment, and software of all descriptions. There are arrangements for individual students to select materials for use and for groups of students to view materials required for a particular assignment. There are computers and software for student use, with much of the software developed by the faculty of the school. Instructors have various informative evaluation tests on computers.

Media Laboratory

The learning center has a well-equipped media laboratory with professional staff to assist faculty in various media productions, ranging from transparencies and slides to video productions of professional caliber. There is assistance for all facets of production, including development of ideas, script writing, decisions about most effective medium, and costs. The staff of the learning center includes a full-time nurse faculty director, nurse faculty, audiovisual and computer media specialists, a librarian, and student assistants. Besides the extensive staffing, equipment, and programs of the learning center, school of nursing personnel have collaborative arrangements with various centers and laboratories in other schools on campus, such as the biomedical laboratories, the university audiovisual studio and center for computer-assisted instruction, the psychology laboratories, and others. The technologies, equipment, and software are continually updated. Just as learning is supported by faculty, library, and clinical facilities, so, too, is it enhanced by a comprehensive learning center that provides instruction through the use of all modern technologies.

CENTER FOR RESEARCH

The center for research exists to promote and coordinate the research activities of faculty and students of a profession that has only recently entered the arena of scientific inquiry. Whereas for centuries research has been assumed to be an integral function for most academicians, members of various practice professions entered the world of academe primarily for the purpose of transmitting knowledge to developing professionals. The focus of their professional functions made it natural for them to enter into community service. For many decades after joining university faculties, they functioned in the two areas of academic responsibilities--teaching and community service. It is essentially only within the past half century that practice professionals recognized that they have a responsibility not only to utilize new knowledge developed by other scientists in their own professional work, but also to engage in studies that would add to the available knowledge. Even today, faculties in some professional schools have limited understanding of the process of scientific inquiry. The center for research is maintained to assist with development of the knowledge and skills needed to engage in scientific investigations.

To fulfill its purpose, the center for research provides many and varied services. Ideally, the center would consist of the entire faculty, and the faculty would make up the center, but since what is everybody's job frequently ends up being nobody's job, it is necessary that there be an established physical entity as well as a concept of functioning. The center is directed by a senior nurse faculty member and has a staff consisting of an administrative assistant, a secretary, and a statistician. In addition, a number of graduate students are employed who possess various research skills in the areas of statistics, computer literacy, development of data-gathering tools, and writing and editing. The center has files of data-gathering tools, a reference shelf of statistics and methodology books, and subscriptions to nursing research and computer journals. There is a suite of rooms, including private offices, for full-time employees, shared offices for graduate students, and rooms to house the computer and word-processing equipment.

Services provided to faculty and students include consultation on all phases of research, data processing, typing, and editing of proposals and reports. Systematic communication keeps faculty members and students informed about research going on in the school, current reports of research in the larger nursing community, funding sources, and deadlines for submitting proposals for funding. A mechanism exists for scheduling presentations by faculty members and students of research in various stages of development, with discussion and criticism by colleagues encouraged. Assistance is provided with development of proposals and interactions with the various individuals and units in the school and university that are involved in the various facets of the research undertaking.

The director and staff of the center assist in planning the assignment and developing space to serve the needs of individual projects. When possible, assigned space is near the center's offices, but frequently it is necessary to use space in other parts of the school. For some studies, space will be contracted for in other buildings on campus, particularly when the study involves collaboration with faculty in another school. The director and staff of the center provide services to graduate students that parallel those provided to the faculty. Research-related services are provided to undergraduate students on a somewhat limited basis, and they receive the majority of their assistance from the faculty members providing their instruction in research.

Funding for the center is part of the overall budget for the school. Money comes from the university administration, from grants obtained by faculty in the school, and from contracts with agencies for doing a particular piece of research. The school advisory committee includes descriptions of activities and needs of the center's program when seeking funds from potential community donors.

The center for research is a major resource in a top-ranked school of nursing, with its services and functions expanding as more faculty members pursue investigations and the number of graduate students increases.

COMPUTERS

The staff, students, and faculty make extensive use of computers. Computers in the student affairs office handle student records and promote student advising and program planning. Administration offices use computers for storage and gathering of information and for word processing. Computers are used to provide faculty with secretarial, typing, and printing services. The learning center has a bank of computers that provide students with computer-assisted instruction and assist in developing computer literacy. Curriculum requirements for classes at all levels ensure hands-on computer experiences. The research center has a number and variety of computers, including portable terminals that can be checked out by faculty and students and line linkages with the mainframe computer in the university computation and data-processing center.

The university has entered into programs with manufacturers to allow faculty members to purchase personal computers at or below cost. Many nursing faculty members have their own personal computers, and discussions are underway to provide a personal computer at each faculty member's desk. Faculty members are using computers for research and for teaching and are developing innovative software for both purposes. They are also developing new strategies for using computers in teaching and are conducting research and evaluations regarding the use of computers in teaching and in delivery of nursing care to patients. Nurses are fully aware of the potential of the technologies to promote various activities related to nursing, and many are actively exploiting the potentials. Both administration and faculty colleagues support expeditious progress in use of computers.

Computers in several of the libraries on campus are available for unlimited use of faculty and students and are not restricted to literature searches. Undoubtedly, computers are the single most useful and used resource to be added to universities and schools of nursing in the past decade.

OTHER DEPARTMENTS OF THE UNIVERSITY

Other Faculty

The nursing faculty view themselves as part of the total university and take advantage of the many opportunities, both planned and incidental, for interaction with other health professionals who are scholars in other schools and departments of the university. They share in decisions and policies that advance the mission of the university. They receive outstanding cooperation from faculty of other schools, whose assistance they seek for their own teaching and research, for consultation to students, and for participation in special programs. In turn, faculties of other schools accord them peer status and seek their assistance in areas of their knowledge, interests, and expertise. Physiologists share research projects; engineers assist with equipment and instrument designs; pharmacists provide updated information in pharmaceutics; nutritionists share patient care planning; economists assist with studies of costs of nursing care.

Perhaps the most frequent interaction is with the faculty of the school of medicine. The two faculties collaborate in planning student learning experiences in the university hospital, arranging joint classes for nursing-medical students, and pursuing scientific investigations of patient care problems. Nursing faculty and students have access to patients in the university hospital for clinical practice and for research. In many investigations, they collaborate with physicians and the nursing services staff in the hospital. Nursing staff and faculty interact extensively on all levels to the benefit of both groups in student instruction, patient care, and research. Such interactions may be casual, but there are also many formal occasions planned to promote their mutual interests. Both small groups and individuals meet regularly; for example, the dean and the director of nursing service meet on a planned basis, as do the faculty coordinator for clinical practice and the nursing staff member assigned as liaison to coordinate student experiences within the hospital. Clinical faculty meet with individual head nurses. All view these interactions as promoting their individual concerns for the profession, for their job responsibilities, and for fulfillment of the missions of the school, the university, and the hospital. Students are involved in collaborative planning for sharing with faculty and students in other disciplines, as well as with other nurses. They develop the habit of thinking about potential for assistance from experts and feel free to consult faculties in other departments in the school and in other schools on campus, as well as professionals in clinical settings.

Courses and Programs

Courses of general interest or needed for cognates by nursing students are readily available throughout the campus. Many departments, including psychology, growth and development, pharmacy, guidance, and economics, welcome nursing students in their courses, not only as a service to the students, but for what the students bring to the courses. In some high-demand courses such as counseling, the school will reserve spaces for a number of nurse students. Some courses are planned and listed as joint courses; for example, in nursing-pharmacy, economics-nursing, ethics-nursing, and primary care nursing-medicine. Nursing students are invited to attend special programs in various schools, and several, including the school of medicine, send them special notices of major programs. Nursing students are kept informed of opportunities to meet national figures.

Another important type of cooperation among schools is the ease with which nurses can gain admission to programs of doctoral study in other schools. Many faculty members are pursuing doctorates on campus.

Equipment and Facilities

Nursing students and faculty have access to equipment in many schools and receive assistance in use of the equipment. They use various laboratories in the school of medicine, including cadaver and other anatomy laboratories. Biomedicine, bioengineering, and nutrition are among the laboratories used by nursing students. Nursing students, faculty, and staff enjoy the use of sports and recreational equipment and facilities, and computer and audiovisual equipment and facilities in other schools are accessible to nursing students and faculty.

Centers and Hospitals

The many specialty centers in the university are all accessible to students and faculty in nursing. Nurses currently take advantage of many of them, but find that they discover new potentials for others as use of familiar ones increases. The university hospitals and the many health clinics are major resources for nursing students and faculty; they are used for instruction and for research. But there are numerous other centers designed to extend competencies of faculty and enhance learning opportunities and experiences for students.

The student affairs office of the university parallels the services of the student affairs office of the school. It provides initial advising information about and orientation to the university; referrals; funding sources; tutoring; and career counseling and placement. In addition to serving students in relation to their careers, the office maintains a file on each student and uses letters in the file to respond to all requests for references, so that a faculty member needs to write only one letter of reference for a student.

Other campus centers with which the student may have contact are the writing skills lab, the counseling center, the student health center, and, of course, the libraries and computer center. Centers that faculty may consult for assistance with their work include the center for teaching effectiveness (all new faculty have a one-week concentrated course as part of their orientation) and the measurement and evaluation center, which provides for course evaluations by students and assists instructors with test development, administration, and grading. A fast-growing, multidisciplinary center is the center for aging whose development is shared by the faculties and graduate students in psychology, social work, pharmacy, nursing, and economics, among others.

Administration

Ultimately, the university administration is responsible for and provides all resources in the university, but some functions seem particularly tied to administration. One important, helpful, and frequently used center is the office for research funding and sponsored projects. As the name implies, that office oversees matters related to research funding--the seeking of funds, their expenditure, and accounting for them. In addition, however, the staff provide other needed services to students and faculty. They share in planning for research awards; know of potential sources of funds; have information about special interests of agencies, organizations, and foundations; and monitor research proposals for the protection of human subjects. Nurses have frequent occasion to consult with staff of that office and receive extensive, interested assistance from them.

FACULTY AND STUDENTS

Faculty are reported by all those interviewed as being the most important resources of the school. Some students' comments illustrate just how important they are:

> The strongest resource is the faculty. Everything goes back to that. If we had to save one thing in a fire, I say save the faculty.

> Faculty is my major resource; they always have current information and latest resources.

> The faculty is the single most important element in making us a top-ranked school.

The faculty continue to grow and increase their contribution as a resource for the school. The nursing faculty are also used by faculties in many other schools as resources for their knowledge, thinking, and planning capabilities.

In turn, students are viewed as resources as well. There is a mix of many attributes within the student body--students vary in age, education, experience, ethnic and socioeconomic backgrounds, interests, goals, and life-styles. There are many international students with whom nursing students have frequent and varied opportunities to interact. The students serve as inspiration and stimulus for faculty innovation and growth, and they serve as multipurpose resources to each other.

STAFF

The quality and support of staff can be summed up in a few brief statements made by students and faculty alike:

> We have a great secretarial staff.

> The secretarial and other support staff feel as affiliated with the school as do the faculty.

> The quality of the staff and support facilities of the school are as great as any in the university; way better than other places.

> The staffs of the various centers--whether professional, technical, or student--make a positive difference. They are always cheerful and helpful.

> There are word processors at all secretarial stations.

> Secretarial assistance is available when needed.

Relationships among staff, faculty, and students manifest
mutual respect, cooperation, and friendship.

Essentially, faculty and students are commenting on the importance of
staff as resources. They report that staff are outstandingly competent
and are provided in numbers and with skills that contribute to expeditious
functioning of people and programs in the school.

PLANT

Many are impressed with the school of nursing's building. It is considered pleasant, comfortable, efficiently arranged, and conveniently located
in relation to other units of the university. A shuttle bus is available to
facilitate transportation throughout the campus and the residential community
of students. Both students and faculty appreciate the security accommodations,
including the presence of a guard during evening hours.

Students also appreciate lounge areas, locker rooms, and ready access to
all areas of the building. They see these facilities as indicating concern
for them, making them welcome, and contributing to high morale. Students are
also pleased about arrangements for them to receive communications through
assigned mailboxes. Graduate students are certain that various facility
arrangements, such as meeting rooms and study carrels, greatly enhance their
sharing, studying and learning accomplishments.

There is flexibility in the assignment and use of space. As size of
student groups and instructional or research projects change, changes are made
in room assignments. Some rooms have movable partitions to accommodate needed
changes in room configurations. A space committee made up of faculty, staff,
and students is responsible for continuing planning and for annual review of
space utilization. Comments indicate that, although they may not be important,
the pleasant surroundings and convenience that the building provides for the
varied study, learning, and social activities make a difference.

ADVISING AND COUNSELING

Many of the elements related to advising and counseling are reported
in the section on faculty concern for students. Rather than repeating that
information here, a few quotations will serve to portray the support provided
students:

Faculty are accessible and available to students.

There is a low faculty/student ratio.

Faculty are willing to listen to students.

There is a commitment made between the faculty adviser and
the advisee from the beginning of the program to job placement.

Faculty make you aware of available resources and how to use
them.

It is easy to get appointments with faculty. They have an
open-door policy. They are available or you can readily
find out when they will be able to see you.

There are many occasions for students to talk to faculty.

The advising relationships in the school of nursing are
widely acclaimed throughout the university, by faculty and
students alike.

There are counselors in admissions to do career counseling.

Student affairs office provides supplemental assistance to
students; they help with many problems.

Students have many resources for advisement and counseling assistance,
with the assigned nurse faculty advisor being the primary resource. She in
turn refers students to the many other resources in the school and university
to extend additional assistance.

PROGRAM FUNDING AND SALARIES

Faculty Enrichment

The dean and, in turn, department chairs allocate portions of their annual
budgets to support faculty attendance at special meetings and programs, either
to present papers or attend as a learner-participant. Endowments, including
professorships and visiting lectureships, support learning opportunities for
all faculty of the school and allow those holding endowed positions time and
money to pursue enrichment experiences to meet their own interests. The
university and the school budget funds to bring experts to the campus and
bring new ideas to faculty and students. They provide opportunities to meet
and talk with famous people. Many faculty members of the school of nursing
are innovative in obtaining funds to advance learning opportunities for
faculty; they share ideas, efforts, and accomplishments.

Salaries

Salaries were seldom mentioned by those interviewed. In many instances,
they either commented that salaries are competitive or that salaries were not
the major element in attracting them to a faculty position at the school.
The latter comment seemed to imply that salaries are low, but that the many
positive attributes in the school compensated. Frequently, the faculty

member's spouse is employed in the university or in the community and is the primary breadwinner. This allows the faculty member to accept what is seen as a desirable position.

Sources of Funding

There are many sources of funds to be used for various purposes in a university. Among the primary sources are state and federal governments. State funds are allotted to support fundamental education programs in the arts, sciences, and, increasingly, in the professions. Funds are provided for basics, such as buildings, equipment, and faculties. For funds for special educational programs and for research, the university must make special budget requests. Universities of renown, both state and private, are apt to receive greater funding than other state-supported schools within any one state. This means that the school of nursing within a renowned university enjoys a high level of funding; it is treated with equity by the university administration.

Federal funding is provided in research grants that are won by faculty, a limited number of research contracts, special educational support grants, and traineeship grants for students. The latter usually support students in programs focused on particular health care concerns, such as maternal-child health or psychiatry. Administrators may develop requests to be submitted for federal funds for traineeships and innovative broad educational programs, such as initiation of a new doctoral program or a new outreach program. Faculty are expected to demonstrate competence in grantsmanship and to develop pro-posals to support teaching programs in special areas as well as their own research efforts.

Besides tax-based sources, funds are available from many private sources, organizations, businesses, and foundations. Many are interested in supporting programs for health care, programs for research, and, increasingly, demon-stration projects to enhance care and increase the availability of indi-viduals qualified to improve health care for particular population groups. For example, the Robert Wood Johnson and Kellogg Foundations have supported programs for nursing homes and for hospice care.

FINANCIAL AID FOR STUDENTS

Tuition

Renowned universities and top-ranked schools of nursing have a commitment to facilitate opportunities for qualified students to enter and complete educational programs in their schools. The university budget includes funds for various needs of students, including tuition, fees, books, and living expenses. The university and the school of nursing have funds earmarked to attract and support minority students. Some students come with scholarships given by private organizations, such as the Elks Clubs; some have National Merit Scholarships; and some have federal fellowships provided for students in the health professions. Both the university and the school of nursing have a fund to provide small emergency loans that enable students to remain and progress in their programs. The various funds are provided in the form of scholarships, loans, and assistantships; students apply through the student affairs offices.

Besides the funds administered by the university, the school of nursing has funds for similar types of assistance to students. Some 50 percent of undergraduate students and a larger percentage of graduate students receive some form of funding through the school during some portion of their program. Besides ensuring educational opportunity for students, the funds enable the school to attract high-quality students from various parts of the country and to particular programs. For example, students are attracted to programs in maternal-child nursing and psychiatric nursing, where specialists are in such short supply that the federal government provides traineeship funds in efforts to attract potential practitioners. Once a student has entered and is succeeding in a program, every effort is made to provide the financial assistance needed to complete the program. The staff in the student assistance offices collaborate closely with faculty to help the student obtain and make judicious use of funds. Research and teaching assistantships for students exist at all levels. Teaching by undergraduate students includes tutoring other undergraduates, guiding junior-level students in the skills laboratory, and assisting international students with the language. Graduate students are assigned research and teaching tasks commensurate with their knowledge and capabilities.

In sum, the types of financial assistance for students are many and varied; they are evidence of a commitment by the school to do all possible to ensure an education to all qualified students who desire one.

CHAPTER 7

SOCIAL CONTRIBUTION

The social contribution of the school includes the individual and collective endeavors of faculty, students, and alumni aimed at improving the
health of society. The top-ranked school has made, and continues to make,
significant contributions to all levels of society: the local community,
the region and state, the nation, and the world. These social contributions
are accomplished through a wide range of activities, such as establishing
nursing clinics and private practices that provide direct health care services,
developing educational programs to meet the health needs of nurses and society,
pursuing scholarly endeavors to increase the knowledge base of nursing, improving the practice of nursing by involvement in professional and health-
related organizations, and effecting needed changes in the health care system
through political and legal activism. All of these efforts have the general
purpose of improving the health of society, with particular attention to the
needs of the poor, elderly, women, and other minorities.

IMPACT ON HEALTH CARE

The school of nursing is an active force in improving the health of the
local community. Faculty and students have identified areas of need and have
established service programs where they provide health care. They work in
soup kitchens, in shelters for the homeless, in programs for immigrant and
migrant families, and in inner-city health clinics. The school of nursing
has initiated many of the health programs that are now being carried on by the
community, such as nursing clinics in medically underserved areas; screening
programs for children, adults at risk, and the elderly; and outreach health
programs for the rural population.

The faculty encourage students to survey the community and identify
services they might provide. Students and faculty explore these areas and
develop strategies to provide the needed health care. As one commented,
"There is a real commitment to society. . . . We want to effect change that
will make society better." Students develop a good understanding of their
community and have experience in the various community endeavors of the
school. Graduates often assume new roles for nursing in the community that
were begun by students.

The school also promotes the health of the community by sponsoring
activities, such as health fairs, CPR classes, blood pressure screening,
supplying needed health information to the public, and promoting consumer
advocacy. Because of the positive reputation of the school in promoting the
health of the community, faculty are often asked by agencies and groups to
provide needed services. Members of the school are asked to be on local
health boards and agencies, develop and implement needed health care services,
offer health education programs, and serve as health care consultants. Said
one faculty member: "Last year we contracted with a county to do a health
assessment for them. This provided a service to them and opportunities for
faculty practice."

INFLUENCE ON EDUCATION

The school of nursing has a major influence on the health education of the community. It is committed to education of consumers regarding their health and their rights to health care. Health education is an integral part of the various services provided by the school.

The continuing education program of the school of nursing provides valuable services to the community. Agencies contract with the school to provide continuing education and to co-sponsor workshops and seminars. The school has contracts with local and state health departments to teach physical assessment to their nurses. Other health care agencies contract with the school to provide classes on management to their nursing personnel. The school also provides continuing education programs to agencies and universities in other countries.

The school continues to be responsive to the educational needs of nurses locally and throughout the state by providing graduate nursing education. Many of the nurses with a master's degree who are working in the community have received their graduate education from the school of nursing. The school has "developed educational programs to prepare nurses for special roles, such as clinical specialists, midwives, and primary care practitioners," and it has developed specialized areas in the graduate programs in response to the needs of nurses and society. Some of these specialized areas include women's health, family health, substance abuse, occupational health, and nursing service administration. "We set the pace for nursing by providing a new wave of leaders so that nursing will in turn set the pace for health care."

IMPACT OF SCHOLARLY ENDEAVORS

The emphasis on scholarly endeavors of the faculty has an impact on the local community as well as the larger society. Nurses in the community are often involved in clinical research projects directed by individual faculty members or the research center of the school. "We contribute new knowledge to this community and to the country. We improve nursing practice by conducting research studies of clinically relevant problems." Through these efforts, nurses and others in the community are gaining experience in the research process, developing an appreciation for the value of clinical research for nursing, and providing better health care to clients.

Researchers in the school of nursing are identifying new fields of nursing science and developing demonstration projects. The school disseminates new knowledge gained from research through many avenues, such as local and state conferences, local and national publications, and consultations to health care agencies interested in conducting nursing research studies. The school has been responsible for initiating the formation of local and regional nursing research groups that collaborate on areas of mutual interest.

In many cases, service programs to the community were originally set up as research projects. After the research study was completed, the service was offered to the community, including an evaluation component. As one participant commented, "The school of nursing is fully committed to serving the community. . . . They strive to communicate research findings to nursing and the lay public."

CONTRIBUTIONS TO THE NURSING PROFESSION

The school of nursing is committed to the advancement of the nursing profession, as evidenced by the various contributions of its members. "Faculty and students are outspoken in promoting nursing. . . . Aggressive advocacy in promoting the nursing profession and protecting the rights of clients."

Faculty and students are actively involved in their respective professional organizations. "Faculty and students do a lot of work at the state and national level to direct the future of nursing." They hold local, state, and national offices in the American Nurses' Association, the National League for Nursing, the American Association of Colleges of Nursing, Sigma Theta Tau, regional and state research associations, and numerous clinical specialty organizations.

The school of nursing plays a significant role in portraying a positive image of nursing through its influence in the university, its involvement in social issues, and its preparation of professional nurses for many different roles in the state and nation. It "plays a part in socializing students into professional roles. . . . They prepare their graduates to be leaders in nursing."

Networking is an important aspect of the school of nursing. The faculty establish networks throughout the state and nation with other faculty members who share common scholarly interests. Students are also "encouraged to establish networks with other nurses so they can contribute to the nursing profession as a whole." Faculty members serve as role models in networking for their students, nurses in the community, and other women.

POLITICAL ACTIVITIES

The school of nursing has made an impact on the political and legal system by its involvement in health-related issues locally, statewide, and nationally. Faculty members contribute by lobbying for bills that are in the best interests of nursing and health care, such as third-party reimbursement, nurse practice acts, and needed programs for minorities and the underserved. The school emphasizes the importance of nursing's involvement with health policy and many of its members are active in politics. They are recognized as leaders in the area by the university and community.

Students and faculty explore relevant health care issues and plan what nursing's contribution will be. Both groups become involved in what needs to be done. It is assumed that "all members of the school have a responsibility to make a contribution to the community." Faculty are expected to be involved in health care legislation and, in turn, they expect students to gain the necessary experience and knowledge to make an impact as professional nurses. Noted one faculty member: "We've developed the social-political conscience of students. Three of our state legislators are nurses and our students work with them." As part of their graduate education students have courses in health policy and practicum experiences with a variety of local and state politicians.

The school has been influential in promoting the rights of women and other minorities. "Our women's health group has helped to promote feminism and women's health in the area," a respondent reported. The school has also been involved in meeting the specific health needs of blacks, Mexican-Americans, immigrant families, migrant families, and the rural population.

CONTRIBUTIONS OF INDIVIDUAL FACULTY MEMBERS

Although all faculty members are involved in some form of service to the community, the following examples will serve to highlight the quality and extent of their contributions:

Federal monies were cut off for rehabilitation programs. One faculty member launched a letter-writing campaign addressed to president and Congress. Funds were restored.

Faculty serve on boards of trustees of various groups: Children's Hospital, college boards, editorial review boards, etc.

Speaking engagements, consultations, publications, participation in university community.

Central and East Africa--faculty consultation produced an education project.

Outside contributions of faculty: League of Women Voters, boards of VNAs, retarded groups, mental health, governor's task forces.

Very involved with state and city government, president of city council interested in infant mortality and I served on a related community board in an advisory role.

Psychological/mental health faculty member got first award for a nurse. Developed an assessment tool, which also has been included in a National Institutes of Health packet.

Pediatric faculty promoted needs of handicapped children--developed parents groups for children with spina bifida--still very active.

One faculty spends one month per year (last seven years) in
Indonesia--clinics.

Teach in high schools, involved in town meetings--do these
on my own but see them as service to community.

Faculty on regional health planning commission. Former
faculty are now in high city and state positions. Director
of state board of nursing--former faculty.

Faculty are alert to direct nursing profession through their
research and publications.

Faculty dedication to profession. One runs home for
battered women. One does a lot of research on birth
control for teens. Doing more than just teaching. Dean
speaks nationwide. Faculty involved in ANA and the state
nurses' association.

STUDENT'S WORK

The social contributions of students are primarily through their work in
clinical agencies in the community, as the following comments illustrate:

Graduate programs contribute to health of citizens of state,
faculty in midwifery run midwifery in county hospital.

Students are change agents in organizations; help redefine
roles in organizations.

Students' work in the nursing home project is a good
contribution to care.

Process and places where students go is an arrangement to
meet societal needs. Give tremendous service to people with
social needs: from ghetto to upper class; rural to urban.

Annual health fair for the community.

Students outsopken in promoting nursing; promote human
values in technological health care sense.

Students in community agencies--our expectations of
students, raises caliber of care in agencies.

Contribution to health of city: student participation in
Health O'Rama, blood pressure clinics. Faculty and students
active in state nursing organizations.

Graduate students address community groups: aging,
disabled; do sex education; have community-focused health
fair every year.

Get involved in policy issues at state and local levels, national levels.

Students and graduates really believe in holistic health and helping.

Help people in hospitals or homes go back to work and into the real world. An extension of our education but a real contribution to society.

INFLUENCE OF ALUMNI

The school has a strong and supportive alumni who have made significant contributions to nursing and health care. Their contributions and visibility locally, nationally, and internationally contribute to the top ranking of the school of nursing. Examples of the support and influence of the alumni are the following:

There is a strong supportive alumni. Many in community serve as preceptors for our students in clinical.

Alumni are very strong; on-going tangible support. People really participate here and in the regions. Regions have their own alumni chapters. They are great public relations people. Alumni feel very loyal to school of nursing. They expect an on-going relationship with school of nursing.

Capable of going into wide range of settings; perform at competent level. Assured leadership positions. Students establish a reputation of clinical competence early, then move on to leadership positions.

Alumni in clinical agencies come to school of nursing, ask us to help plan and develop care practices; these are then available to faculty and students.

Socialization into high level of professional awareness. Frequent contact with alumni. Breakfasts with alumni and students at national meetings. Alumni on advisory committees in school of nursing.

Qualified graduates--reflection of curriculum and faculty. BSN graduates very highly valued by employers, and they tell us this. Good reputation that students are well prepared.

We have graduates in every state in the United States except Nebraska.

Our alumni also make us top ranked--several have been deans. It seems that we have been and are a training ground for deans. They moved to all parts of country.

A continuing leadership in nursing and health care. Alumni have started BSN programs in other countries (France, Nigeria, etc.). Continually work with minorities. Leaders improving access to health care for all.

Alumni serve in underserved areas--urban, rural, jail.

Reputation of our BSN program--highly sought by military. Graduates take responsible positions.

Very active alumni association. Alumni activities well attended. Networking is phenomenal. Alumni seek each other out at national meetings, etc.

Doctoral program's graduates have added to the positive image of nursing in general, and nursing in particular areas such as the military nurse.

Doctoral graduates have taken . . . research facilitator positions in hospitals; some are co-directing funded scholarly projects.

Networking; graduates of doctoral programs are visible throughout the United States.

Our graduates are willing to take risks in their employing institutions and people listen to them.

Our graduates have never had any trouble getting jobs.

People leave the program wanting to go on for more education--turned on to education. Also sense that it is possible to do it--facilitates a "go for it" attitude.

CHAPTER 8

POST-INTERVIEW COMMENTS

Immediately following the group interview, participants were asked to complete a written Post-Interview Comments Form (Appendix D). As noted earlier, these post-interview comments allowed respondents to describe their ideas about what might be. The rationale for including this portion of the study was that despite the many positive elements of the school discussed in the interview, most respondents would also have ideas about how it might be improved. Many might have suggestions or even well-thought-out plans about how improvements could be effected. In relation to the study, these ideas had the potential to provide still further descriptions of components of a top-ranked school. There was also the possibility of gleaning ideas for future developments in nursing education.

All participants were asked to respond in writing, within a 30-minute time period, to the following challenge:

> If unlimited and continuing funding were made available, along with the stipulation of full functioning within two years, describe a proposal that you would make for a change or innovation to be established in your school within this time period.

The ideas were as varied as the individuals proposing them. They were organized into nine major categories, with an accounting of the number of proposals in each category. The frequencies in each category were distributed about equally among the five groups of respondents; for example, of suggestions about curricula, 11 were from administrators; 20 from senior faculty; 12 from junior faculty; 9 from graduate students; and 14 from baccalaureate students. The categories, along with the numbers of proposals in each, were the following:

Support for research	25
Nurse-run clinics	14
Curricula	66
Organization	4
Computers and technology	11
Collaboration with nursing service	10
Plant, equipment, resources	13
Student needs, e.g., transportation	11
Listings without plan details	37

Just as for other information gleaned in the study, a summary will not serve readers; only the limited number of responses that would not be expected to provide ideas for program improvement will be summarized. A few responses focused on a problem peculiar to the individual school and could be expected to have little or no generalizability to other schools. In a second group were proposals for actions that would provide an advantage or desirable situation for faculty or students, but would be unlikely to affect the quality of the school's programs. In a third group, a number of responses were limited to listing suggestions of changes or innovations, with no delineation of programs to effect them. The foregoing account for about 30 percent of the responses. All others presented ideas that could be useful for planning.

The authors did the difficult task of selecting from the nearly 200 suggestions, 24 that might provide ideas for students, faculty, and administrators. An attempt was made to avoid personal biases: included are proposals that one or more of the authors may not favor. A single criterion guided the selection: Is implementation likely to enhance the quality of a program of a school of nursing? When titles were assigned to identify the focus of each proposal, it was found that the selected proposals could be listed more appropriately in categories that differ from the original organization. The proposals are presented as they were written, with very limited editing, along with deletion of school identification, in one or two of them. They are presented in the sequence of the new list of categories: (1) endowment, (2) curriculum, (3) teaching strategies, (4) nursing care of particular populations, (5) health policies and social issues, and (6) research.

The reader is reminded of the constraints under which the respondents wrote. They had just complete a two-hour group discussion where free interchange and informality were encouraged but where many challenges to serious thinking were posed. They were then asked to settle down to identify an idea and delineate a plan for its implementation in writing, all in 30 minutes. From the limited number presented here (and many times the number were worthy of presentation), it is obvious that respondents seriously addressed the task. The expressions of the ideas are adequate for others to grasp, and the plans for implementation, although brief, are adequate to serve as a basis for planning by any interested group.

ENDOWMENT

With $5 million I would establish three chairs at $1 million each. The available funds from these endowments would be used to provide student fellowships, research funds for faculty, travel funds for professional meetings, and supplement to salary of the holders of the chairs.

Additional professional endowments would be established, and on a smaller scale would do the same as chairs.

I would establish three visiting professorships which would support the established visiting professor program.

I would establish lectureships which would pay for visitors for faculty development in a variety of areas.

From one of the endowed professorships I would use funds to further expand ane enhance the Regional Center for History of Nursing.

CURRICULUM

Undergraduate Curriculum Revision. There is enough evidence in current nursing literature (Styles, Hipps, Pardue, etc.) that the "integrated" curricula in nursing are causing "globalization" and confusion of nursing's essential content. Students are being confused by ambiguous concepts, multi-syllable conceptual frameworks, and complex nursing process paper work. Much of what students learn in the undergraduate curricula is "meaningless" to them as they enter the real nursing world, whose language and functional syntax is different from nursing education's to some extent. I believe that nursing education needs to be revised in our own undergraduate curriculum in order to offer relevant knowledge and skills pertinent to today's and tomorrow's nursing and health care demands reflected in the real world.

We have some evidence (research based) from assessments of our own graduates that there is need for curriculum change. Although curriculum change is somewhat painful, it can be handled with expertise if the appropriate faculty are appointed to head a revision team and given the time to facilitate the process.

It seems essential that we utilize the knowledge, strengths, and talents of faculty in the most effective curriculum we can. The current one does not seem to reflect the best combination of essential content, course organization, teaching assignments, etc.

International Exchange

Development of the International Nursing Program. Strengthen the relationship with other schools in other parts of the world where this school has an existing relationship, by developing a center for international studies with faculty who are expert in international health and nursing and who have an interest in it. Facilitate student and faculty exchange programs with other schools outside the United States. American students and faculty would conduct research in other countries (cross-cultural research) to validate the tools and theories that they have developed here. Faculty would teach in different settings and learn about the consultation process. International students and faculty would come here and learn, and participate in the school's activities. The establishment of this center could be facilitated with collaboration with the World Health Organization's nursing division. Through this center, graduate nursing students from the U.S. who are enrolled in this school could gain learning experiences (clinical, teaching, research, consultation) in other countries, so this center could prepare American nurses who are specialized in international nursing, and who could contribute to nursing internationally.

Seminars and courses pertaining to international nursing and cross-cultural research could be effected through this center. There are schools in the U.S. which are opening divisions for international nursing and need prepared faculty or administrators to direct these divisions. Graduates of this school who have gone through the activities of the international nursing studies center could be potential candidates for these positions.

More Research in BSN

I propose that a program be developed in which undergraduate students become more active in happenings at the university's center for health research. Although this is available at the senior level as an elective, I feel a required exposure to research activities in the undergraduate program would promote growth of the students and improve the caliber of graduates from the school.

I propose the program as follows:

1. Students complete the Introduction to Research class in the first semester of junior year.

2. During the following semester, students are assigned to current projects based on preference.

3. Once assigned the students begin participating in the projects: collecting data, analysis of data, footwork for the researchers. The time involved would be about 2-4 hours weekly.

4. At the end of the semester, the student has the option of continuing research involvement through the summer and following year for credit.

5. The funding for the program would cover cost of the student tuition for the course and provide a monthly stipend.

Not only would the student benefit from experience in the practicum, the researchers would gain help in the project, and the university would have graduates at the baccalaureate level with experiences like those of master's students.

Physiology

Our school is well equipped to teach research and provide service to patients whose needs are psychosocial or psychophysiological in origin. We have the clinical laboratories for study in this area. What we lack at the present time are the resources for study of phenomena from a perspective which is primarily physiological. Thus, the basic research to answer questions which nurses may want to aks cannot yet be conducted with ease in this setting. We are moving toward it. But if I had unlimited funds I would secure the necessary laboratory space and a critical mass of nurses with PhDs in physiology and nurses with PhDs in nursing with a physiological emphasis to establish research programs and secure funding in their area. I see this as the one needed area of development in our program at this time. We're working on it, but lack of funds really is the problem!

Transcultural Nursing

I would propose an almost all (95%) doctoral facility in order to develop a top-level consortium to rigorously pursue explication of nursing in unique and distinct nursing knowledge and to develop ways to verify the use of the knowledge in new modes of health care. This consortium-like research institute would be developed with care and health as the dominant domains of inquiry and with a strong transcultural nursing focus. This proposal would focus on comparative health systems and the majority of systems (or social structure elements) would be new innovations in making nursing a distinct, compelling, and attractive discipline and profession to the world. Our traditional health care systems are no longer viable, and it is time for nursing to take a leadership role in nursing education and service to initiate some entirely new modes of health care. Concomitantly, it is time for nursing to introduce new curricular changes based upon research and theory, and to make nursing a fully respected discipline. A transcultural approach to this proposal would give the new, exciting direction for nursing's future.

Outreach: Midwifery

Proposed: Expand the Nurse-Midwifery Curriculum to the Regional Sites

1. Assist the development of nurse-midwifery practice sites in other areas (one now operating, two others possible soon). The process involves education of the public and health professional in those areas and demonstrating how they would benefit from our services; also practical help in writing protocols, etc., and work at the state level on reimbursement mechanisms.

2. Since funding would be available, persuading the faculty and administration of the desirability of the proposal probably would not be a problem.

3. A task force of current faculty with participation by regional site faculty would design the curriculum.

4. We would advertise nationally for a PhD-prepared nurse-midwife to coordinate the new program. (This should probably be done early, because it will not be easy to achieve. However, being able to offer a handsome salary makes the task much easier.)

5. Facilities such as office and laboratory space, teleconferencing and computer facilities would have to be developed. It would not make sense to repeat all courses in each area, so teleconferencing would enable students there to participate in courses from the school.

6. Clinical faculty appointments would have to be arranged for staff certified nurse-midwives in the clinical facilities.

7. Advertise that the program is available!

8. Use our experience as a model for other nurse-midwife programs in the country to expand.

(This is just off the top of my head. I'm sure it would be more complex then this. However, plenty of money does smooth the way.)

Mentorships in Residency

Since I have benefited enormously from being actively involved with my mentor in several research projects during the last half of my master's program and throughout my doctoral program, I feel this should be a requirement for all doctoral-level students. I feel that a formal structure could be set in motion whereby this could be accomplished. At the beginning of doctoral study, students would be informed as to the types of research projects ongoing or to be implemented. They could then select a project most attuned to their interests. This could serve as a research internship during which students would gain both didactic and practical experience regarding all the various facets of conducting research. Project directors could monitor the experiential exposure to ensure a wide variety of experiences. This range of experiences would include: literature review preparatory to proposal development, proposal writing, getting through IRB procedures, negotiating clinical site arrangements, instrument development, actual data collection, data reduction and analysis, report preparation and dissemination. Such an arrangement would facilitate the incorporation of an active and practical research orientation into whatever career path the student would pursue post-doctorally. The essential element in such a structure, of course, would be mentors who would provide guidance and leadership for such research internships. Junior faculty could also be incorporated into such a structure as project directors. In this way a network of various groups functioning at different levels of sophistication could be implemented and nurtured.

Computer Course in BSN

With unlimited funds and the emphasis placed on computer operation now, a course should be developed and required to make BSN students computer competent. The ability to work with comfort in relation to data retrieval systems could promote research in the hospital environment and gain added respect for the value of BSN graduates. Relatively simple program operations could be taught that allowed leeway for individual computer systems.

Examples for use could be the itemized: nursing budget with exact amount for certain types of patients, percentage of nursing resources used in each unit and where, balance amount of patient education to return admission for similar diagnoses, and show the overall efficiency of nurses versus support staff specialists (i.e., respiratory therapists, heart-lung technician, etc.). Many occupations today require personnel to be "computer-friendly" and those who are will have the advantage or at least equality.

The most difficult part of this program would involve the focusing of the student on the benefit for the patient for this information. The computer must not separate the nurse and patient but allow more efficient patient contact with techniques and even more time for education of the patient.

TEACHING STRATEGIES

Computers for Teaching Learning

Proposal: To modernize the school of nursing by introducing on a large scale computers and computer programs. In order to stay in competition with nursing and other disciplines, this is essential. By incorporating computer technology into nursing, all aspects of health care would benefit; i.e. clients, education, and nursing research. Clients would benefit from the findings of research in health care and the increased availability of facility to meet the needs of both students and clients.

Through the use of computers in education, computer programs could be established individually for nursing programs at the BS, MS, and doctoral levels to facilitate nursing education. On the research level, data collection and analysis would be expedited, and therefore greater qualities of research could be done.

Implementation of this project could be accomplished in two years by the following:

-- Obtaining experts in the computer technology to help select equipment.

-- Training faculty to use computer and develop unique computer programs.

-- Requiring courses in computer science for students and faculty.

-- Developing doctoral program which allows the option of writing a unique computer program for nursing as a doctoral thesis option.

Interdisciplinary Team for Patient Care

Utilize the medical center environment, polling of the resources of various schools, i.e., medicine, pharmacology, dentistry, etc. Possibly go on rounds with medical students to help develop rapport with physicians; learn how to give input with regard to patient care and treatment. This would help potential nurses learn the rationale for measures taken by the various health care team members. Also incorporate longer exposures (or possibly a rotation) in OR. At present you only get a week. I feel this type of experience would augment the student nurse's socialization into "real hospital life" when he/she enters the working world upon graduation. It would also facilitate the development of a more positive outlook toward team work with all members of the health care team. Since the nurse has the greatest length of (and more personal) contact with the patient, I feel this teamwork approach could help the physician, pharmacist, etc. as well as the nurse.

Joint Faculty Services: School of Nursing-University Hospital

I feel we are working toward this goal. I would like to see the University Hospital become a laboratory for trying out new, innovative ways of nursing practice, incorporating faculty, students and staff. The goal would be to have an outstanding hospital (home-health care, clinics, HMO included) where nursing is operational at the highest professional standards of practice. It would translate to optimum patient care around the clock. Primary nursing would be totally operational (not just talked about).

Students would therefore be exposed to excellent role-modeling. The PhD-prepared faculty would collaborate with master's prepared clinical leaders and nursing staff in research aimed at improving patient care and developing the scientific basis for nursing practice.

Within this model, the students of any level (undergrad, master's, PhD) could independently work on a research project, could select a variety of courses for elective hours (e.g., critical care nursing, perioperative nursing, advanced med-surg clinical practice, etc.). Nursing would collaborate with other disciplines, e.g., pharmacy, dietary, physicians on joint research projects. This would be an increase in nurse-run clinics (we have one already). There would be greater emphasis on preventive care, home health care, geriatric care, women's health care, etc.

BSN minimum level would be required to be hired by the hospital. Criteria required of head nurses would include master's degree in nursing, competence in nursing practice, and demonstrated leadership; could hold PhD or DNSc. University hospital would hit the top-ten list for excellence in nursing practice.

Joint Appointment/Collaboration

With a rapidly changing society, educating students to apply new concepts and ideas in the "real world" can be problematic if students do not have access to a mentor relationship with a skilled teacher-clinician. There is a clear need to move toward utilizing clinicians in various agencies as preceptors for students and to create a program that helps the clinicians to expand their knowledge and conceptual base. Movement toward this objective would require the development of an administrative mechanism--headed by an interested faculty member--to negotiate arrangements with the participating agencies and to work out a program plan that would probably include special seminars, faculty serving as mentors for clinicians, and various give-and-take activities.

The first year would be a planning year--and would involve establishing a specific focus, organizing details of who would participate from faculty, negotiation with the agencies, and working out the mutual participation activities.

Second year would be a trial run of the collaboration arrangement. Hopefully, clinicians could be exposed to new ideas, research results, etc., and faculty could be exposed to the various real problems of nursing care.

All of this would depend on interested faculty, employment of support people, and some creative thinking. The results would be a shift in working arrangements between school and clinical agencies.

NURSING CARE OF PARTICULAR POPULATIONS

Adolescent Health

A Program of Adolescent Health. Specifically: fund a center to do more work in the areas of adolescents, 1985:

-- their needs

-- their pressures

-- problems related to single parenting

-- either their own parents or parenting themselves

While the proposal would initially be health oriented, it would evolve into studies that would address issues of

-- adolescent parenting

-- adolescent suicide

-- adolescent addicting abuses

Staffed, of course, by experts in the field, to train/educate health care professionals and provide services to the region.

Women's Health

Center for the study of nursing phenomena, such as women's health. This center would support a cadre of faculty concerned with problems related to women's health; it would support a faculty practice clinic, ongoing investigations of several problems women experience across the life span, testing nursing protocols for these problems, pre-doctoral and post-doctoral training of investigators, and master's and baccalaureate students' practice experience. Such a center would promote the integration of scholarship, teaching, and practice; preparation of clinicians and investigators; and make a major contribution to the health of women in this community.

Research Center: Multidisciplinary Center on Aging

I would propose an interdisciplinary research center devoted to issues of chronic illness and aging. We already have a complement of faculty and doctoral students committed to these areas on a small scale and a center on aging in the university, but both suffer some of the constraints that inadequate funding imposes. In a sense this is not a true innovation, since the seeds are here currently, but in another sense it would be a real change because it would promote and facilitate the interdisciplinary approach that needs to take place if real progress is to be made in the health care of the elderly. Lack of funding has forced the center of aging to be only concerned with certain service functions, which inhibits its ability to collaborate with other departments and schools interested in research on aging issues. I believe nursing and especially our school of nursing has the human resources to make a real contribution to improving health care to the elderly.

Additional funding would help us to widen our scope and extend our efforts further and eventually establish nursing as a leader in health care for the elderly. The two years' full funding would release key people to devote full time to operationalizing the concept of interdisciplinary research.

HEALTH POLICIES AND SOCIAL ISSUES

Health Policy

Proposal: To initiate a Center for Health Policy within the School of Nursing.

Implementation Process: With the dean's knowledge and expertise in health policy, this institute could be initiated without difficulty, given the release of restraint of funding. The center could give impetus to policies pertinent to nursing to demonstrate nursing's contribution to the health of society. A group of highly knowledgeable individuals could easily be recruited for such an endeavor.

In order to accomplish this, we need resources for strong task groups to map out total plan involving faculty experts along the way and the administrative support to expediently move the changes through the system; etc., etc., etc.

Health Policy Studies: Interdisciplinary

Goal: Establish a formal Center of Health Policy Studies which is housed at school of nursing but involves interdisciplinary participation-- similar to health policy/administration centers at Northwestern, Vanderbilt, Minnesota, etc.

Method:

1. Identify a health policy research project which is sufficiently interesting to attract health policy interests across campus.

2. Work in interdisciplinary team to develop proposal for:
   a. campus research board
   b. national funding source

3. Begin pilot project work in interdisciplinary team.

4. Involve graduate students in project to allow their experience to help group to begin identifying discrete subprojects that provide for individual recognition for each participant.

5. Complete pilot project.

6. Continue major proposal/study work.

7. Formalize study group via institutional membership in association of health services research.

8. Continue group activities to develop reporting/sharing sessions for discussing project results, new ideas for future projects, etc.

Minority Students

As we increase the number of minority students in the School of Nursing (Black-American, Native Americans, Spanish surnamed and Spanish speaking, and Asian), I would like to provide a counselor specifically for minority students to increase the retention of the ones now enrolled, and to continue to recruit those not now represented (Native Americans and others). Counseling, currently, is provided by the Office of Student Services and by the Minority Affairs officer who carries a full academic load. The ratio of students to counselors is too great to allow adequate time needed to advise students with specific or multiple problems. A start-up program for a short period could perhaps lead to a way to more effective counseling for recruitment and retention.

Minority Students

The most beneficial improvement I could propose would be the establishment of an aggressive affirmative action program for both faculty and students. Access to institutions of higher education for ethnic minorities is a continuing problem in this society (grown worse in the last few years) that is reflected in the student body composition of this university in general and this school in particular. Our experience and training have demonstrated that few things change for the better without careful assessment, planning, implementation, and evaluation.

Nursing outreach/recruitment programs should begin in high school and continue during the first college year. Support services/programs should be included to assure retention and graduation of such recruits Even prior to this, someone (committee, task force, etc.) needs to ask why more minority students/faculty are not here--Are they rejected due to poor grades or lack of qualifications? Do they choose other schools? Do they choose other careers? Are they under economic constraints?

Faculty recruitment of minorities is also important. They can provide valuable role models and, hopefully, an "inside" perspective on minority communities and some of their unique concerns.

Social Issues

Establish a center for the study of social issues in nursing. It would be composed of humanistic pairs:

Philosopher -- Nurse ethicist

Economist -- Nurse economist

Historian -- Nurse historian

Anthropologist -- Nurse anthropologist

Political scientist -- Nurse expert in public policy analysis

Others

They would focus as a think tank to deal with overall issues; then they would pair up for study of issues of particular interest to them or of current social concern.

RESEARCH

Research Institute

I would see established an institute for nursing research. I would use the funds to recruit more seasoned researchers to this campus and to offer them the supports they need to pursue their scholarly work. We have the positive, supportive atmosphere, but we need on board statistical experts and more easily available access to computers and computer troubleshooters who can take some of the pain away from statistical manipulations/interpretations that we now feel. We need more funded research assistants/scholarship help for graduate assistants in these roles. We need secretarial/duplication resources that are more available/reliable than those in place at present. We could use some easier access to some health care institutions to be receptive to research by nurses, and perhaps funding would make their cooperation more assured; i.e, we could assure them that allowing the study would cost them nothing and perhaps the school could reimburse them for access to their client populations through offering inservice education to their staffs, tuition reductions to their staff, etc.

With financial supports to increase the research efforts of this school I'm convinced magnificient work, in abundance could be done, judging from the quality of the effort/production that has been evidenced when we work with so little.

Research Focus for School of Nursing

I would like to see areas of concentration for faculty research and graduate study identified and developed. Such areas would focus faculty research efforts and give direction to recruitment activities. Achievement of this goal would require the following:

1. Identification of areas of concentration which cut across departmental boundaries (e.g. family, women's health. This would probably entail a series of faculty forums or retreats).

2. Recruitment of faculty with ongoing research in area to complement our own current faculty.

3. Recruitment of students (graduate) into areas of concentration.

4. Seed monies for developing courses/research in areas of concentration.

Research Focus for School of Nursing

Full state-of-the-art technology implementation in research and communication to the extent that the focus on the technology is subsumed under the rubric of scholarship and developing the science of nursing (i.e., so the focus shifts to uses of the tool for professional purposes and not on the tool itself).

The process should include:

-- Planning with participants and consultants.

-- Hardware and software acquisition.

-- Implementation, including instruction/evaluation/revision.

-- Final evaluation.

Concurrently, I would foster development of research focus groups interested in pursuing like/similar areas of nursing science so that content and process would develop together--drawing in outside expertise as required.

CHAPTER 9

CONCLUSIONS AND RECOMMENDATIONS

It is expected that as individuals and groups use the information compiled in this study, they will consider its meaning for a particular school. Each school is as unique and complex as that profiled in the report. It may be expected, therefore, that people using the report will interpret the meaning of any of the findings in light of the reality in the school of their concern. Nonetheless, broad conclusions can be drawn to identify various highlights of the profile of a top-ranked school of nursing.

1. A top-ranked school is a complex organization, with integrated functioning of many elements.

2. The school can never be static; change is a constant reality.

3. A school is composed of many individuals, each with diverse interests and expertise.

4. The dean is a strong, knowledgeable nurse administrator.

5. The school employs qualified personnel, who have:

   -- Support and freedom to pursue their own interests and to individualize their practices.

   -- Opportunities to develop and grow.

   -- Responsibility for their primary concerns--teaching students, research, curriculum, and quality of nursing care.

6. Student are satisfied with the programs; they believe that faculty are accomplishing the professed goals of the programs.

7. Administrators, faculty, and students weave perceptions about research into descriptions of all components of a school of nursing, most especially when talking about the dean, faculty, and curricula.

8. The school has the same autonomy accorded all other schools and colleges of the university.

9. The school makes notable contributions to the health and welfare of the local and regional communities.

10. Resources are varied, they derive from many sources, and they are efficiently used to provide for the many programs of the school.

RECOMMENDATIONS

The type of recommendations usually associated with study findings and interpretations would be prohibitively numerous for this study. Determining the actions suggested by the findings and interpretations will be left to those who use the report to plan changes in their own particular situation and program. The authors do, however, recommend some general uses for the report and materials used in the study:

1. When read with a particular school, program, or area in mind, the report can serve as an evaluation guide.

2. For beginning planning, the total report should be reviewed. There are so many interrelationships that many ideas would be missed if reading were limited to selected portions.

3. The interview schedule and process can be used with various groups in any school to serve two purposes:

   a. To identify perceptions about components, processes, and interrelationships in a school.

   b. To inspire positive thinking and excite persons about their own programs and school.

Support for the latter recommendation derives from statements made frequently by members of all groups of participants. One dean commented:

> It was fun to "blow our own horn," something we seldom have opportunity to do. In fact, I would say that it was therapeutic.

Two assistant professor noted:

> All faculty should participate in such an exercise. It would help all of us to become more aware of how good things really are.

> Thank you for the opportunity to seek out many positive attributes of our school. We don't take enough time to do this.

Baccalaureate students were enthusiastic. To quote again the student cited as the outset of the report:

> I never before have spent two-and-one-half hours discussing only positive things--about anything. It is really a wonderful experience.

A senior student at The University of Texas declared:

> This was so exciting. For the past three months, what with the pressures of completing my degree requirements, I have done nothing but gripe about everything. Now, I see it completely differently. I shall leave happy!

APPENDIXES

Appendix A

Planning for Data Collection

THE UNIVERSITY OF TEXAS AT AUSTIN
School of Nursing
Austin, Texas 78701-1499

December 17, 1984

Dean's Name
School of Nursing
University
Address
City, State, Zip

Dear .... :

This letter is pursuant of our telephone conversation during the week of
December 3, 1984, for the purpose of formalizing planning initiated during
that call. As you know, The University of Texas at Austin School of Nursing
will conduct a nationwide study designed to identify factors that make up top-
ranked schools of nursing in the United States. A copy of the abstract of the
proposed study is enclosed. The study will be done by faculty of our school.
Dr. Mabel A. Wandelt will serve as the principal investigator, and Drs. Betsy
Bowman, Mary Duffy, and Susan Pollock will share responsibilities as co-project
directors.

The plan for the study is an analog of the American Academy of Nursing's
Magnet Hospital Study. Essentially, the proposed study will do for top-ranked
schools of nursing, and for all schools of nursing, what the Magnet Hospital
Study did for magnet hospitals and for all hospitals: provide a description
of the elements that constitute a high-quality program. Dr. Wandelt was one
of the four-member task force that conducted the Magnet Hospital Study. The
mechanics for that study were done in our Center for Health Care Research and
Evaluation, with Dr. Wandelt guiding the work, analyzing the data, and writing
first drafts of the report. This background makes her eminently prepared to
guide the proposed study.

Six schools have been selected randomly from the 20 top-ranked schools of
nursing identified by Dr. Patricia Chamings in her recent article in Nursing
Outlook, September/October 1984. Your school has been selected as one of the
six schools, and I am happy that you have agreed to participate in the study.

I have enclosed several attachments which delineate the particular involvement for you and others in your school. Details for the data collection, including identification of groups, scheduling, and arrangements are presented in these enclosures.

Because of possible influence of information contained in the abstract on some responses to interview questions, we are asking that you not share the abstract with others until April 1985, when we expect all data will be collected.

Instead of the abstract, we are supplying you with copies of an Information for Participants sheet that you may give to each person as you invite them to participate in the study.

I know only too well that what I am asking requires considerable effort on the part of you and your staff. I too am going through the process of scheduling the various group interviews for the pilot study which will be done here in mid-December. I do believe, however, that the results of the study will be of great value to all concerned with education for nursing. And of course, success can be maximal only with contributions from yours and similar schools. You will note that we are asking you to make the various arrangements, but we shall provide payments for the costs of luncheons and morning and afternoon refreshments, as well as for all expenses of our visiting faculty.

We have scheduled the interviews with groups from your school for _____, _____, _____, _____, and _____ morning, _____. Dr. Duffy and Dr. Pollock will maintain telephone communication with you or your designate, as needed, to establish agreed upon schedules and arrangements for the visit to your school for the data collection interviews.

I firmly believe that many of the positive, important things taking place today in our top-ranked schools of nursing have not received the attention that they merit. The time has come to identify what factors are integral to high-quality schools of nursing. I also believe that such information about programs and experiences within exemplary schools can be of great assistance to many educational programs throughout the United States. For these reasons, I thank you for your participation in this project.

Please contact me or Dr. Wandelt if you have any questions associated with your decision to participate. We can be reached at the following number: (512) 471-7311.

Sincerely,

Billye J. Brown, RN, EdD, FAAN
Dean
LaQuinta Motor Inn, Inc., Centennial Professor

Attachments

The University of Texas at Austin School of Nursing
Top-Ranked Schools of Nursing Project

Responsibilities of Deans or Their Designates

The dean is asked to make the following arrangements:

1. ### Selection of Group Members

   Six members are to be invited for each of the following groups of persons knowledgeable about their school:

   -- Dean, associate or assistant dean(s), department heads;
   -- Full professors and associate professors;
   -- Assistant professors and instructors;
   -- Graduate students (master's and doctoral); and
   -- Baccalaureate students.

   Inform invited person about the purpose of the study, assuring them that participation is voluntary. They should also be informed at this time that their choice not to participate will not hurt their relations with the school.

   Provide a copy of Information for Participants about the study and interview session (Attachment I) to each of the 30 members who agree to participate. Schedules of the 30 members will have to be coordinated to permit participation in the appropriate group.

2. ### Scheduling of Group Interviews

   Schedule five 3-hour group interviews; they may be scheduled in any order during the 3-day visit. Fill in the identity of groups on the agenda to indicate the order in which groups have been scheduled (Attachment II). Two copies of the agenda should be provided to the interview team on its arrival at your school.

   Complete a list of participants for each group (Attachment III), which includes their names and primary assignments. Please have two of these lists of each group for the interview team at the time of their arrival at your school.

3. ### Scheduling Room for Group Interviews

   Schedule a room on the premises that has a large table (or table arrangement) and eight comfortable chairs. The arrangement should be such that the eight persons may be seated comfortably facing others around the table, with table space for writing materials.

   There should be a side table for refreshments.
   Please provide a scratch pad and pencil for each participant.
   Please prepare a place card for each participant.

4. Scheduling Luncheons and Refreshments

Arrange a luncheon for all participants on each of the three interview days, from 12:00 noon to 1:00 p.m. Due to limited time, the lunch should be provided on the premises. If needed, lunch may be in the same room as the interviews. On Day 1, the lunch will include only members of the first group. On Days 2 and 3, there will be a single lunch for both morning and afternoon groups.

Arrange for refreshments for the group participants throughout each morning and afternoon (coffee and soft drinks).

5. Hotel Reservations and Directions for Travel

Arrange hotel reservations for the following nights: _____, _____, and _____.

Two single rooms will be needed for the research team. Provide directions for the research team about sources of ground transportation from airport to school, hotel to school, and hotel to airport.

6. Communication

Communicate with the research team if you need to clarify your understanding of planning for the group interviews and preparations needed. The names and phone number of the research team are: Dr. Mabel A. Wandelt, Dr. Mary E. Duffy, and Dr. Susan Pollock; (512) 471-7311.

7. Responsibilities During Three-Day Visit

Share hostess responsibilities with research team during the three-day visit.

ALL EXPENSES FOR ACTUAL COSTS OF LUNCHEONS AND REFRESHMENTS, HOTEL, TRANSPORTATION, AND SUPPLIES WILL BE ASSUMED BY THE RESEARCH TEAM.

The University of Texas at Austin School of Nursing
Top-Ranked Schools of Nursing Project

ATTACHMENT I--INFORMATION FOR PARTICIPANTS

You are invited to participate in a study about top-ranked schools of nursing. The purpose of the study is to delineate the elements that comprise top-ranked schools of nursing. Your school is one of the six top-ranked schools that was randomly selected for this study. Although your dean has approved participation of your school as one of the six schools selected, your participation in the group interview is voluntary. Your decision whether or not to participate will not influence your present or future relations with The University of Texas at Austin. A Participant Consent Form will be given to you to read and sign at the beginning of the group interview.

There will be five group interviews in each of these six schools. Each group will be made up of five or six individuals from the following categories of persons: deans and their assistants; professors and associate professors; assistant professors and instructors; graduate students (master's and doctoral); and baccalaureate students.

You will be a member of one of the groups interviewed from your school. The interview will take approximately three hours, and no preparation will be necessary. You will be given an interview schedule at the beginning of the interview, and these questions will serve as stimuli for the session. Two faculty researchers from The University of Texas at Austin School of Nursing will serve as interviewer and recorder for each session. At the end of the session, you will be asked to complete in writing a brief Post-Interview Comments Form.

Your group will consist of five other _____.
It is scheduled to meet:

                    Day _____

                    Date _____

                    Time _____

                    Place _____

A luncheon will be provided for your group from 12 noon - 1:00 p.m. on the day of your interview.

If you have any questions between now the time of the interview, you may contact your dean or designate who is coordinating the arrangements for your school, or myself. I appreciate your participation in this very worthwhile study.

                    Dr. Mabel A. Wandelt, Professor Emeritus
                    and former Director, Center for Research
                    School of Nursing
                    The University of Texas at Austin

University of Texas at Austin School of Nursing
Top-Ranked Schools of Nursing Project

ATTACHMENT II--AGENDA FOR VISIT

Monday	Tuesday	Wednesday	Thursday	Friday
Date _____	_____	_____	_____	_____
Date _____	_____	_____	_____	_____

School of Nursing: _____

Coordinator: _____

The University of Texas at Austin School of Nursing
Top-Ranked Schools of Nursing Project

ATTACHMENT III - GROUP PARTICIPANTS

Group #_____, Deans and other Administrators

Name & Title   Primary
                                                teaching area or major

1.

2.

3.

4.

5.

6.

The University of Texas at Austin School of Nursing
Top-Ranked Schools of Nursing Project

EXPENSES FORM FOR PARTICIPANT SCHOOLS

School: _____

Please record all expenses that you have incurred as a result of participation
in the Top-Ranked Schools of Nursing Project in the appropriate categories.

Luncheons   _____

Refreshments   _____

Supplies   _____

Xeroxing   _____

Miscellaneous (please list)   _____

TOTAL   _____

At the conclusion of the visit to your school, please give one copy of this
completed form to the research team.

Thank you!

The University of Texas at Austin School of Nursing
Top-Ranked Schools of Nursing Project

PUBLICATION OF MATERIALS

Besides information and opinions expressed during the interviews, it is expected that it will be useful to include in the report of the project some of the materials developed in various schools of nursing.

Your signature indicates that you understand that materials you have supplied the project researchers may be included, in whole or in part, in the published report of the project, and that you agree to have it so used.

Signed _____
                    Dean

_____
School of Nursing

_____
(City, state)

_____
(Date)

You do _____ do not _____ agree to having your school of nursing named as the source of the materials.

Signed _____
                    Dean

The University of Texas at Austin School of Nursing
Top-Ranked Schools of Nursing Project

PARTICIPANT CONSENT FORM

You are invited to participate in a study about top-ranked schools of nursing. The purpose of the study is to delineate the elements that comprise a top-ranked school of nursing. You were selected as a possible participant because you are a member of one of these schools. You will be one of approximately 180 persons participating in the study.

If you decide to participate, I or one of my research associates will ask you to be part of a group interview with approximately five other persons from your school. The interview will last about three hours, and the only possibility of experiencing any inconvenience on your part will be the time involved. You will be given a set of questions at the beginning of the interview. The questions will serve as stimuli for the session and as guides to ensure coverage of pertinent areas of discussion. No preparation is required for the participants. You and other members of the group will be asked to respond to the interview questions. Two faculty researchers from The University of Texas at Austin School of Nursing will serve as interviewer and recorder for each session. At the end of the session, participants will be asked to complete in writing a brief Post-Interview Comments Form. You will be part of a national study that will provide useful and timely information to all individuals concerned with the quality of today's schools of nursing.

Confidentiality of the participants and schools will be maintained during and after the study. Data collected from all institutions will be analyzed to develop a composite of top-ranked schools of nursing. Direct quotes of individuals will be identified only by group category, not by individual or school. Comparisons of responses of groups will be make only between total groups for all schools. No comparisons between groups within the same schools or between schools will be made. A complete report of the findings will be supplied to each participating school to be made available to all participants.

Although your dean has approved participation of your school as one of the six schools selected for the study, your participation in the group interview is voluntary. Your decision whether or not to participate will not influence your present or future relations with The University of Texas at Austin. No risks to any of the participants of the study are anticipated. If you decide to participate, you are free to discontinue participation at any time without prejudice: just let me know. Likewise, your participation may be terminated without your consent.

If you have any questions, please contact me. My phone number and address are at the bottom of the form. If you have additional questions later, you may contact me any time during the study. You are making a decision whether or not to participate. Your signature indicates that you have read the information provided above and have decided to participate. You may withdraw at any time without prejudice after signing this form should you choose to discontinue participation in the study.

Dr. Mabel A. Wandelt, Professor Emeritus
and former Director, Center for Research
School of Nursing
The University of Texas at Austin
1700 Red River
Austin, Texas 78701
Office: (512) 471-7311

....
_____   _____
Signature of Participant   Date

....
_____   _____
Signature of Investigator   Date

Appendix C

Interview Schedule

SUGGESTIONS FOR FUTURE USERS

The interview schedule was tested during the pilot study, and the decision was made to use it in the same form for the total data collection. Based on more extensive use of the schedule, the authors propose four changes to be considered by others who may decide to use the schedule:

1. In Question 3, insert "and remain" following "to become," to read, " . . . to become and remain a part of the school?"

2. Restructure Question 6 to read: "What are particular benefits for students in your school of nursing?"

3. Reverse the order of Questions 5 and 6.

4. Restructure Question 7 to read: "Please identify highlights of the various curriculums that warrant top ranking for your school."

Because respondents will say they do not understand questions or that these are difficult questions to answer, there may be temptation to change some of the other questions. But encouraging them to respond in terms of "what you think it means," will start the discussion and lead to full involvement. Essentially, the purpose of the small-group interview and the questions is to get people to think. It is not necessarily meant to be easy.

The University of Texas at Austin School of Nursing
Top-Ranked Schools of Nursing Project

Interview Schedule

1. What makes your school a top-ranked school of nursing?

2. Will you identify and describe a single aspect of your school that you consider a major element in your school being cited as a top-ranked school of nursing?

3. What two or three things about your school influenced you to become a part of the school?

4. What are the outstanding positive aspects about organization and administration of your school?

5. What are the outstanding aspects about the faculty in your school of nursing?

6. What elements in the program(s) for students contribute to the top-ranking reputation of your school of nursing?

7. Please identify highlights of the (a) baccalaureate curriculum, and (b) the graduate curriculum, in relation to:

   (1) the goals of the program(s);
   (2) the mission of the school; and
   (3) the value to students.

8. Please discuss two or three elements of resources and facilities that have major influences on the quality of the program(s) of your school.

9. Other than education of students, please describe the major social contribution of your school, including the personnel and processes that affect the contribution.

Appendix D

Post-Interview Comments Form

SUGGESTIONS FOR FUTURE USERS

It was obvious from some of the responses that one particular part of the challenge was misunderstood by some persons. The intention was that the proposed program would be seen as an ongoing program with continuing unlimited funds. The stipulation of a two-year start-up period was an effort to provide respondents with some boundaries for their ideas. However, some read it to mean that funding would be available only for the two-year period. We suggest that deleting the final phrase, "within this time period," might have lessened the misunderstanding.

The University of Texas at Austin School of Nursing
Top-Ranked Schools of Nursing Project

POST-INTERVIEW COMMENTS FORM

Group ....   School ....
    Please Print   Please Print

You and your colleagues have identified, described, and discussed many
elements and processes that interact to make up the composite that is
perceived as warranting a top ranking for your school. It is accepted that
top ranking is neither attained nor secured by pursuit of the status quo. We
are asking yhou now to highlight an ambition for your school by responding to
the following statement:

    If unlimited and continuing funding were made available, along
    with the stipulation of full functioning within two years,
    describe a proposal that you would make for a change or
    innovation to be established in your school within this time
    period.

DATE DUE

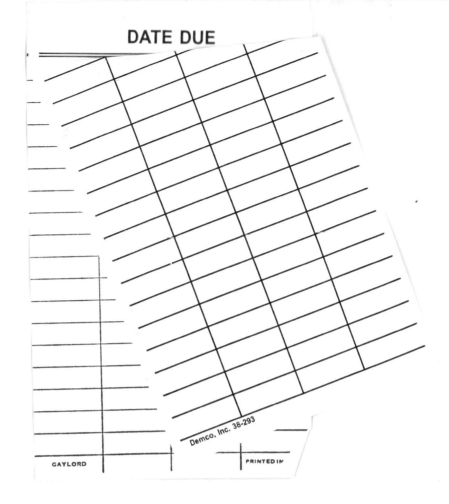

GAYLORD

Demco, Inc. 38-293

PRINTED IN